have your

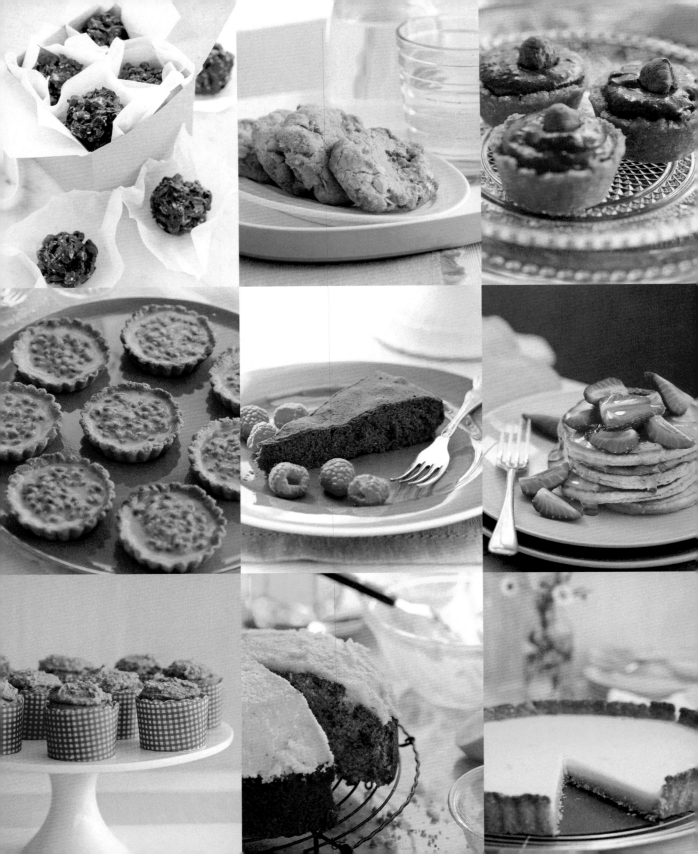

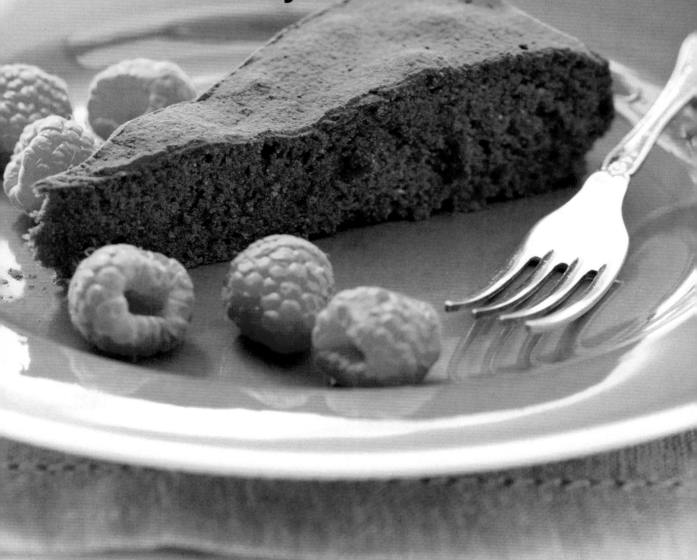

have your cake

a healthy and simple way of baking

no butter • no white flour • no added sugar

emily rose brott

First published by The Five Mile Press, 2011

Second edition published by Emily Rose Brott, 2012
P.O. Box 87 Malvern Vic 3144, Australia
Contact at www.emilyroserecipes.com.au

Cover and page design by Shaun Jury
Photography by Greg Elms
Food styling by Fiona Hammond
Typeset by Sunset Publishing Services Pty Ltd, Brisbane, Queensland, Australia

ISBN: 9780646576688

Some recipes include ingredients that can cause allergic reactions, such as nuts and eggs. If you or your child has a food allergy or intolerance, please check all ingredients carefully and make substitutions where necessary. This book contains recipes that use 70% dark chocolate which contains sugar. However, no recipe calls for the addition of refined sugar.

foreword

Wholesome goodness is what food should be. Cooking at home creates a bond within families, it enhances exposure to different foods and guarantees greater control over the ingredients you consume. With this in mind, using natural, less processed and whole ingredients ensures you and your family receive foods that are as close to their original source as possible and therefore retain a high concentration of nutrients.

Food can be enjoyable and healthy as well, as long as the nutrients have not been lost in processing. Many packaged foods use ingredients that have been modified and contain additives to increase the flavour, colour and shelf life of the product.

With so many different products on the market, it is difficult to know what is best. The allure of the recipes in this book is the use of natural produce and healthy ingredients as opposed to commonly used options. For instance, white flour is replaced with wholemeal (wholewheat) flour, sugar with honey and butter with rice bran oil. Other ingredients with health benefits are also included, such as oats and dark chocolate (70%), making this book suitable for today's foodies.

We know that saturated and trans fats increase the risk of heart disease and many other conditions that are now becoming epidemics; however, replacing these fats with mono- and polyunsaturated fats lowers these risks. Rice bran oil is a 20% saturated fat product, compared with butter, which has 54% saturated fat. As well as its low saturated fat content, it has no trans fats and is high in both mono- and polyunsaturated fat. Rice bran oil also has a high smoke point of 254°C (480°F); this is the temperature at which the oil begins to break down in flavour and nutrition. So rice bran oil can be heated to a high temperature without ruining the quality of the food.

What about sweetness? Sweetening baked goods with sugar improves the food's flavour but has no health benefits. Research shows that sugar plays a role in obesity and its complications, tooth decay and the way we absorb the food. Sweetening food with honey is a better option. Honey, such as yellow box honey, is a natural sugar, and it is much sweeter than sugar, so you don't need as much to achieve the same level of sweetness. The glycaemic index (GI) of honey is also lower than that of sugar, which means that honey is absorbed into the bloodstream more slowly than sugar, having a more gradual and controlled impact on the body.

Regarding GI, when grains are milled and refined (such as white flour) the fibre content is lost, which can increase the GI. Fibre is very important for many bodily functions and, with all the processed foods on the market, we certainly don't eat enough of it. Using wholemeal (wholewheat) flour instead of white flour provides a higher concentration of fibre and keeps vitamins, minerals and phytonutrients in baked food.

Many readily available ingredients are used to improve the flavour of food in the recipes in this book. Chocolate is one of those foods that makes you salivate. Dark chocolate (70%) can be a guilt-free functional food due to the flavonoids present, and high cocoa content chocolate may have the benefit of improving blood vessels, blood pressure and platelet activity.

The more aware you are of the possibility of substituting ingredients to maximise health without changing the taste or texture, the more comfortable you will feel about what you are putting in your body and the bodies of those you are cooking for. The good news about the health benefits of certain foods keeps piling up. So cooking can still be fun, food can still be tasty and the body will certainly thrive!

Joanna Shinewell
BA/BSc (HON) MND
Consultant Dietitian

contents

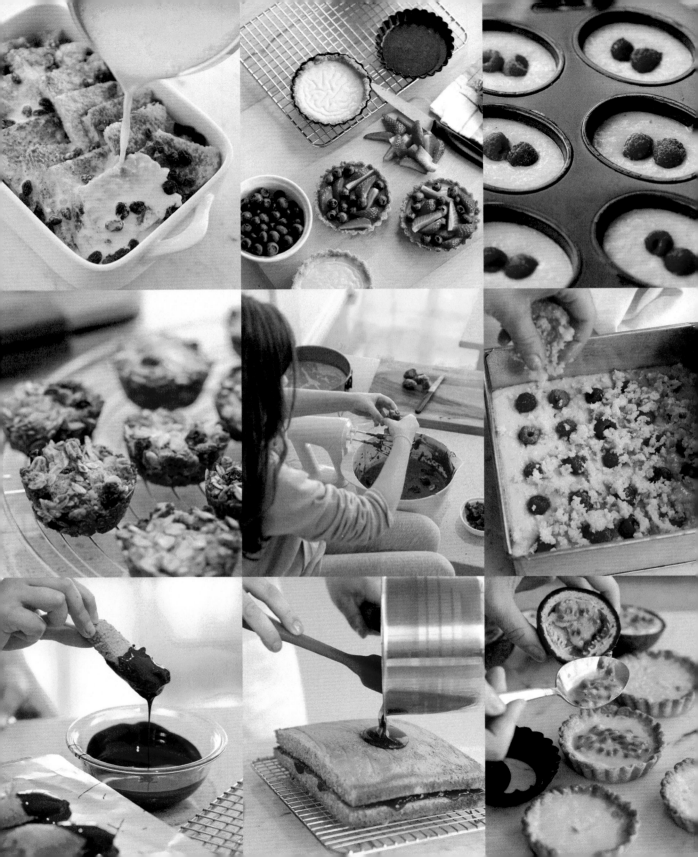

introduction

After constant searching for healthy treats for my children, reading labels on the back of packages of food full of additives, preservatives and lots of sugar, I realised that the best way to ensure that my children were eating foods full of goodness was to bake them myself.

However, I didn't want to just make healthy snacks that looked 'healthy' and tasted 'healthy'. I wanted my children to be able to enjoy treats that looked and tasted like 'normal' biscuits, cakes and desserts, but were made from healthy ingredients.

I also wanted to be able to make snacks that were made from a variety of ingredients that I could keep in the pantry and were accessible from any supermarket.

After visiting a health retreat, and hearing once again about the negative effects of sugar in our bodies, I began experimenting, baking healthy and delicious snacks that the whole family could enjoy without the use of added sugar, artificial sweeteners, butter, margarine or white flour.

Baking and tasting new foods has been a wonderful experience that my children and I have enjoyed together. I was amazed that they began tasting and snacking on the ingredients I placed on the bench while I was preparing the recipes, like dried figs, organic apricots and, of course, dark chocolate. When they began scraping the leftover mixture from the bowl while I was cooking, I knew that the recipe was going to be a success. I also provided samples to our extended family and our friends; they became my test tasters.

The recipes are easy to make and most take only 10 minutes to prepare. I'm often making cookies after I've put the kids to bed.

I hope you, your family and your friends enjoy these recipes as much as we have.

Emily

ingredients to keep in your pantry

rice bran oil*

An extremely light oil, which is trans fat–free, contains vitamin E, antioxidants and nutrients. It also has a very high smoke point so it is great for cooking at high temperatures.

honey (yellow box or raw honey)

Honey is a natural sweetener that provides the body with lots of energy. Yellow box honey has a low GI and raw honey is a pure, unprocessed honey so it retains all of its vitamins and nutrients.

wholemeal (wholewheat) self-raising and wholemeal (wholewheat) plain flour

A great source of fibre as the whole grain is used in the process of making wholemeal (wholewheat) flour, whereas in white refined flour the bran and the germ are extracted.

eggs (use 58g eggs)

Eggs contain high-quality protein and essential amino acids, vitamin E and naturally occurring vitamin D.

desiccated coconut

Contains lauric acid, which may have antimicrobial properties.

almond meal

A source of vitamin E, protein and calcium.

LSA (linseed, sunflower and almond meal)

Contains good fats, fibre and vitamins.

* In Australia and New Zealand rice bran oil is available at supermarkets. In the USA rice bran oil is available in speciality markets, health food stores and online.

oats
Rich in soluble fibre and a good source of many nutrients such as vitamin E and iron.

sunflower seeds
Full of healthy fats, protein, fibres, minerals, vitamin E and other nutrients.

organic dried apricots
Free from sulphur dioxide, which may cause allergic reactions.

sultanas
A good source of energy.

70% dark chocolate
Contains antioxidants.

walnuts
A source of protein, fibre, B vitamins and antioxidants such as vitamin E. High in omega 3 fatty acids.

pecans
Rich in protein and antioxidants. A good source of vitamins and minerals such as iron, vitamin D, vitamin E, vitamin C, folate, calcium and many other nutrients.

10 baking tips

When baking it's always important to follow exact measurements, otherwise your cake or biscuit will not turn out correctly. When people open the oven door to find their cake has flopped it's often because they have adjusted the quantities in some way – such as using a drinking cup instead of a measuring cup when measuring out ingredients. The following tips will ensure success every time and make the baking process easier and more enjoyable for you.

1. Use two separate measuring cups, one for dry ingredients and one for wet ingredients. If you measure the honey after the rice bran oil, it will slide out easily.

2. When measuring flour or other dry ingredients, tap or gently bang the measuring cup on the bench so that all the air pockets in the ingredient are filled. If the recipe says three-quarters of a cup then measure exactly to that line on the cup. One cup is 250 ml.

3. For tablespoon or teaspoon measurements, always use measuring spoons and not your dinnerware spoons. In Australia, one teaspoon is 5 ml and one tablespoon is 20 ml or 4 teaspoons. (Some tablespoons overseas are 15 ml or the equivalent of 3 teaspoons.) Measure teaspoons and tablespoons flat, not heaped.

4. Always grease tins using some paper towel to spread the oil all over the base and sides of the tin. For cakes and friands, line the base with baking paper to make it easier to remove the cake later. Use one-third cup capacity, 12-hole muffin tins.

5. Allow cakes to cool for at least 20 minutes in the tin before removing and leaving to cool on a cake rack. If the recipe suggests leaving it in the tin to cool for longer, then follow the guidelines so that your cake doesn't crack in the centre. Always go around the edge of the cake with

a blunt knife to loosen it from the tin before flipping it out. You can also flip the cake out onto one cake rack and then place another cake rack on top, then flip it over. Leave friands to cool completely before removing from the tin.

6. Place biscuits and muffins on a cake rack 10 minutes after removing from the oven.

7. If the recipe uses honey, always make sure it is dissolved in the wet ingredients before adding the dry ingredients.

8. When using vanilla bean seeds or orange rind, to avoid having a big clump in your mixture, use the back of a spoon to rub the ingredient against the side of the bowl until it begins to break up and dissolve.

9. When melting chocolate, pour some water in a saucepan and place the chocolate in either another saucepan or a heatproof bowl on top, making sure that the water in the saucepan below doesn't touch the bowl above.

10. Always check your cake with a skewer at the end of the set time to make sure that it is cooked inside. All ovens cook differently so it may need 5 minutes more than the time indicated in the recipe. The skewer doesn't always have to come out clean. It can have a little mixture on it as long as it looks and tastes cooked. If it's still runny then cook for another 5 to 10 minutes. If you don't have a fan-forced oven, bake at the temperature indicated in the recipe, but please note that biscuits and muffins may need up to 5 minutes longer and cakes up to 15 minutes longer than the cooking times indicated.

making pastry

To prepare the pastry place plain flour and, where required, self-raising flour in a bowl.

In a separate bowl mix oil, honey and eggs together. Stir in either the orange rind or vanilla bean seeds depending on the pastry recipe. (To extract vanilla bean seeds, slice bean lengthways and scrape out seeds.) Using the back of a spoon rub orange rind or vanilla bean seeds against the side of the bowl until it breaks up and dissolves into the egg mixture. Then add milk.

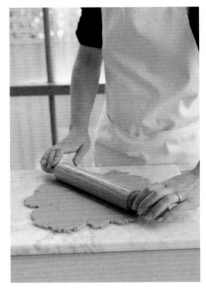

Make a well in the centre of the flour and pour in honey and egg mixture. With a blunt knife gently mix until a dough forms. If needed, place some wholemeal (wholewheat) plain flour on the bench and gently knead the dough until it comes together, then begin to roll out the pastry until it's as thin as it can be without breaking.

Grease tins with oil and cut the pastry into squares that are slightly larger than each tin. Place the pastry over the tin and press it into the tin until the whole surface is covered with the pastry. With a knife or your fingers, break off any excess pastry. If using a large tart tin or pie dish, you may also find it easier to cut the pastry into sections and use your fingers to make sure the edges of the pastry pieces are joined once they are in the tin. Make sure that there are no holes in the base of the pastry, to prevent the filling from leaking.

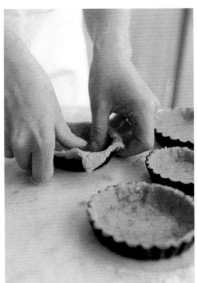

Once you have filled the tins with pastry place them in the fridge for 20 minutes, then 'blind bake' pastry for 10 minutes at 200°C (390°F) to stop the pastry from expanding. To do this, cut out some baking paper, making sure it fully covers each tin so the pastry isn't exposed. Place uncooked rice or baking beads on top of the baking paper and place in the oven. After 10 minutes remove the baking paper and rice or baking beads and let the oven cool to 160°C (315°F), before placing the tart or pie back in the oven for a further 5 or 10 minutes as indicated in the recipe. (To cool the oven quickly, leave the oven door slightly open for a few minutes.)

Fill tart or pie while pastry is still hot to prevent the mixture leaking from the tart shell.

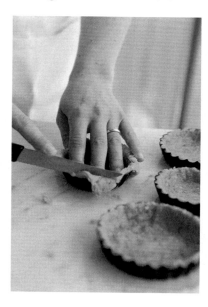
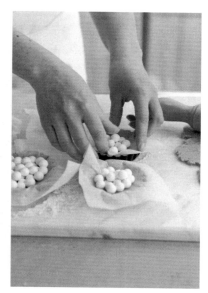

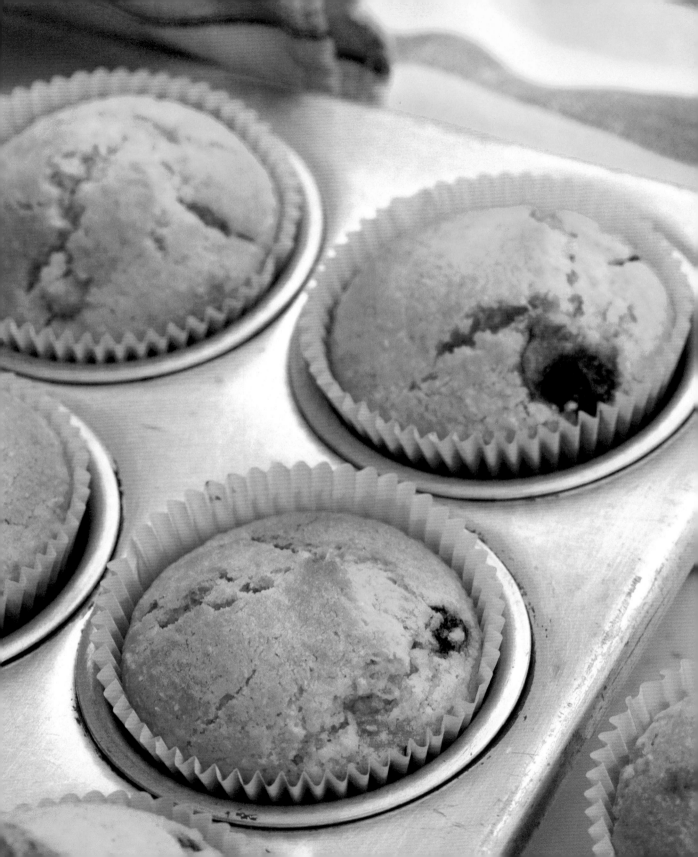

breakfast treats

Eating a delicious breakfast is a great way to start the day.

We like to save these breakfast treats for weekends when there's no rush and we can have breakfast a bit later. Even though most of the recipes only take 5 minutes to prepare, on a busy weekday morning it's hard to find an extra 5 minutes.

Breakfast is a great time to get the kids involved in cooking, whisking the pikelet mixture or preparing smoothies. I always find that the more involved they are in the preparation, the better the treat will taste to them.

I like to serve these breakfast treats with fresh fruits.

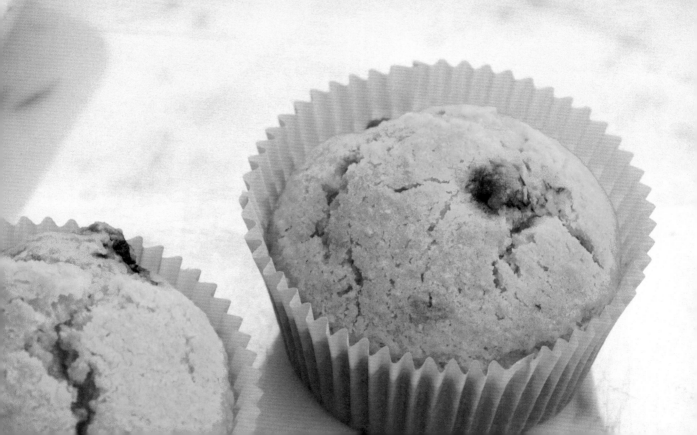

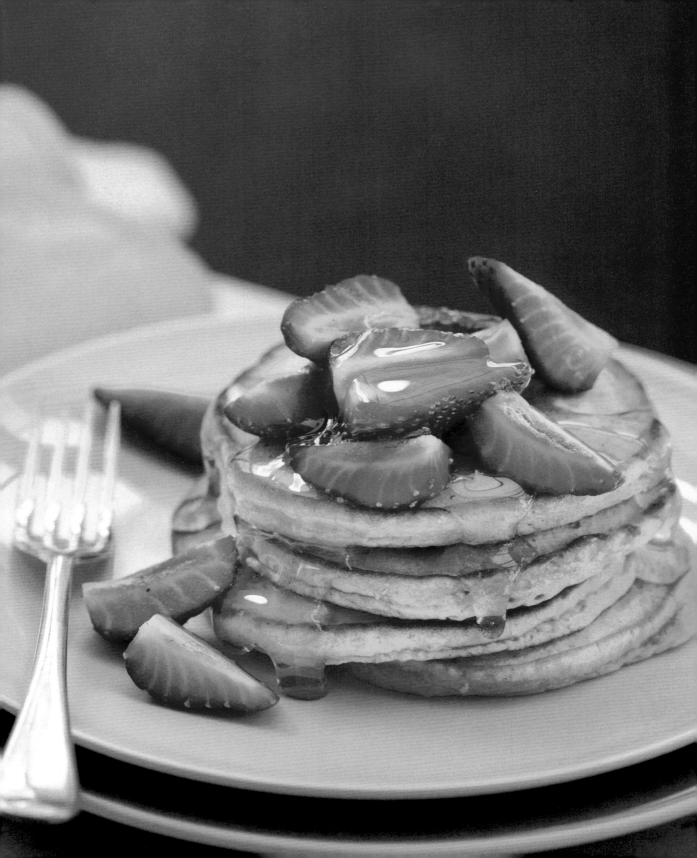

pikelets

ingredients

1 egg

2 tablespoons honey

2 teaspoons rice bran oil, plus extra
for frying

1 cup (160 g) wholemeal
(wholewheat) self-raising flour

¾ cup (185 ml) milk

Mix together egg, honey and oil. Add flour and stir until the mixture is smooth, then stir in milk, a little at a time.

Drizzle a small amount of oil into a frying pan on medium to high heat and pour heaped dessert spoons of mixture into the pan. When bubbles begin to appear on the surface of the mixture, turn pikelets over and allow them to brown on the other side.

Serve them plain or drizzle with honey and serve with berries or your favourite fruits.

Hint: After the first batch, I wipe the frying pan with some paper towel and oil it again. Turn the heat down to low so that the pikelets don't get too brown; the honey tends to make them brown quicker.

crepes

ingredients

2 eggs

2 teaspoons rice bran oil, plus extra
for frying

2 teaspoons honey

½ cup (80 g) wholemeal
(wholewheat) plain flour

¾ cup (185 ml) milk

Whisk together eggs, oil and honey. Add flour and whisk until as smooth as possible. Add milk a little at a time and whisk until mixture is smooth.

Place a small amount of oil in a small frying pan on medium heat. Pour in some of the mixture, moving the frying pan around to spread the mixture so that it covers the base of the pan and isn't too thick. Each side will only take 1 to 2 minutes to cook. Use a spatula to flip the crepe.

Serve with fresh yoghurt and sliced mango.

french toast

ingredients

6 slices rye bread

3 eggs

½ cup (125 ml) milk

rice bran oil for frying

honey to serve

2 bananas to serve

Slice rye bread to your desired thickness. I like it about 1 cm in thickness.

Whisk eggs and milk together. Dip each side of the bread into the mixture twice.

Drizzle a small amount of oil into the frying pan and add bread in batches, frying each side until it is brown.

To serve, drizzle with honey and top with sliced banana.

Serves 3.

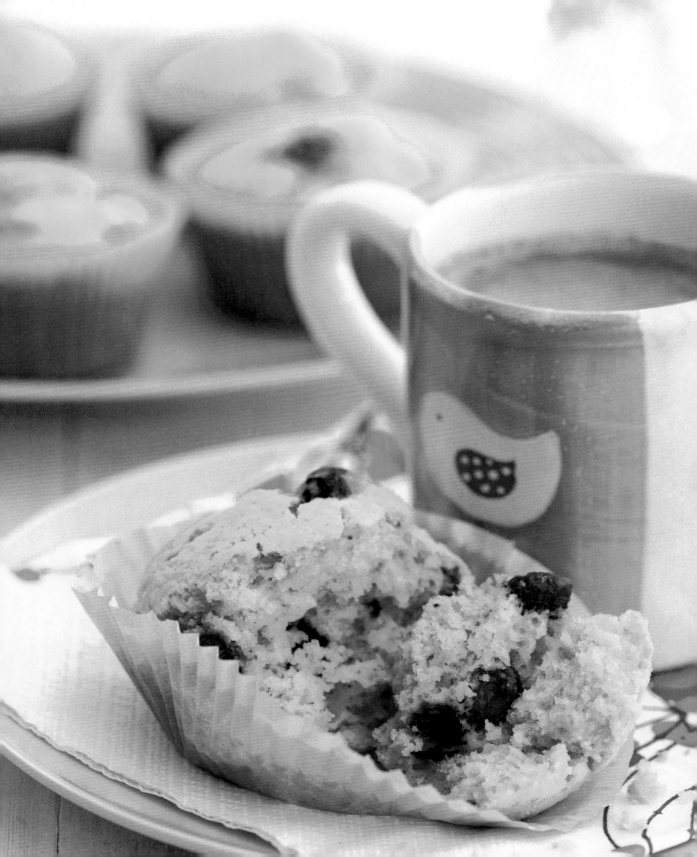

blueberry muffins

ingredients

2 eggs

½ cup (125 ml) rice bran oil

½ cup (150 g) honey

2 tablespoons orange juice

½ cup (50 g) desiccated coconut

1½ cups (240 g) wholemeal
(wholewheat) self-raising flour

½ cup (125 ml) milk

⅔ cup (80 g) blueberries (fresh or
frozen)

Preheat oven to 170°C (335°F) fan-forced.

Using a whisk, beat eggs and oil together, then mix in honey. Add orange juice and coconut. Mix in flour and milk a little at a time, and then gently fold in blueberries with a spoon or spatula.

Grease a muffin tin with oil to prevent muffins sticking. Fill each case ¾ full.

Bake for 20 minutes.

Leave to cool in the muffin tin for 20 minutes. Remove muffins and place on a cake rack to cool further.

Makes 12.

toasted muesli

ingredients
5 cups (500 g) rolled oats
1 cup (140 g) sunflower seeds
1 teaspoon cinnamon
½ cup (150 g) honey
2 tablespoons boiled water
1 cup (140 g) sultanas

Preheat oven to 160°C (315°F) fan-forced.

Mix rolled oats, sunflower seeds and cinnamon together. Stir honey and water together until honey is dissolved. Add honey mixture to dry ingredients, mixing thoroughly.

Line a tray with baking paper and bake muesli until golden, approximately 25 to 30 minutes. Toss mixture a couple of times during baking so that it browns evenly. Once muesli has cooled, toss through sultanas.

Serve with yoghurt and fruit or milk.

banana smoothie

ingredients

2 ripe bananas

1 tablespoon honey

2 tablespoons natural yoghurt

1 cup (250 ml) milk

Blend bananas, honey and yoghurt together. Slowly add milk until all ingredients are blended together.

Serves 2.

Hint: Use a hand mixer or blender to blend the ingredients.

strawberry smoothie

ingredients

250 g strawberries

1 tablespoon honey

2 tablespoons natural yoghurt

1 cup (250 ml) milk

Blend together strawberries, honey and yoghurt. Slowly add milk until all ingredients are mixed together.

Serves 2.

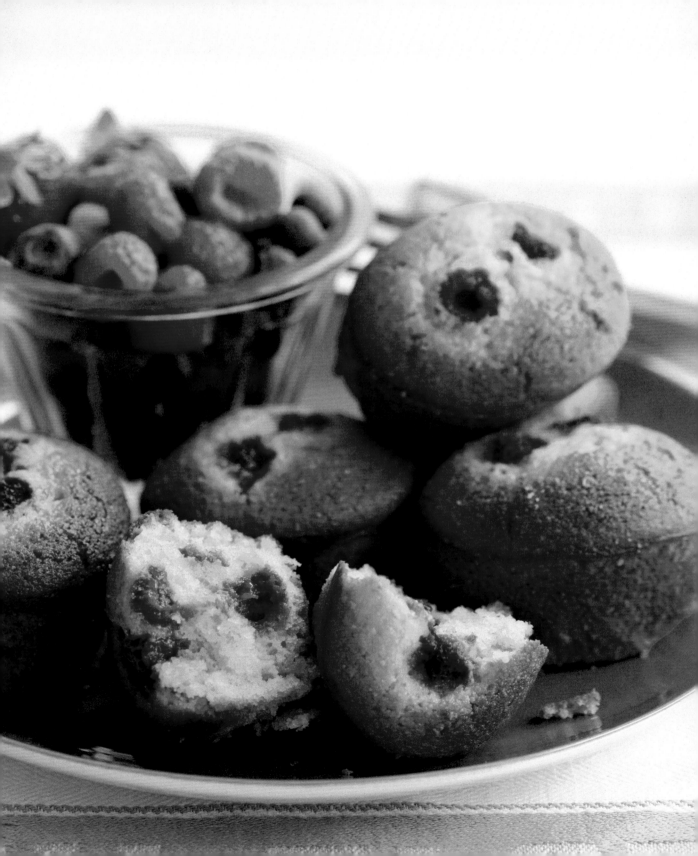

raspberry friands

ingredients

4 egg whites

½ cup (125 ml) rice bran oil

½ cup (150 g) honey

1 tablespoon lemon juice

1 cup (110 g) almond meal

½ cup (80 g) wholemeal
(wholewheat) self-raising flour

32 raspberries (4 for each friand,
fresh or frozen)

Preheat the oven to 160°C (315°F) fan-forced.

Whisk egg whites until fluffy and bubbles have formed on the top. In a separate bowl, mix oil and honey until honey is dissolved. Add to egg whites. Mix in lemon juice and almond meal. Add flour and whisk for a few minutes until the mixture thickens (it will still be a little runny).

Grease a friand tin well with oil and cut oval shapes out of baking paper to place on the base of each case to

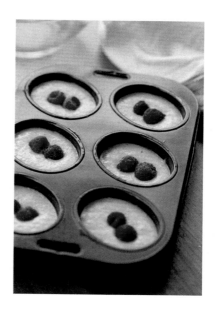

prevent sticking. Pour in mixture, filling each case ⅔ full. Press 2 raspberries into each friand, and leave 2 raspberries resting on the top.

Bake for 30 minutes or until golden; they should feel springy to touch.

Leave to cool completely in the tin.

Run a knife carefully around the edge of each friand to help lift them out.

Makes 8.

Hint: If using frozen raspberries, don't leave them to thaw before using them.

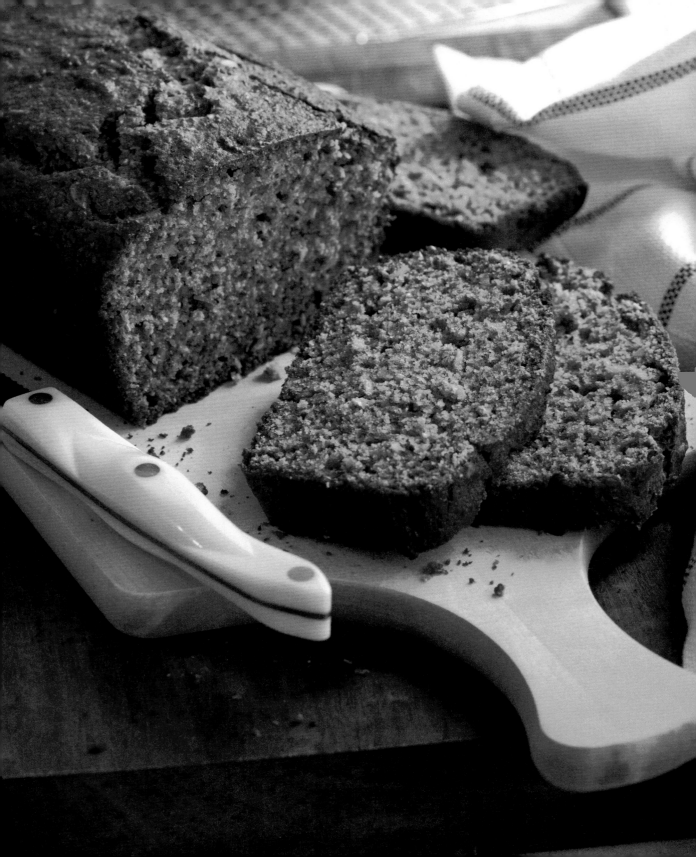

banana bread

ingredients

2 eggs

½ cup (125 ml) rice bran oil

¾ cup (225 g) honey

1 teaspoon cinnamon

1¼ cups (290 g) mashed banana
(approximately 3 bananas)

1¾ cups (280 g) wholemeal
(wholewheat) self-raising flour

½ cup (55 g) LSA (linseed, sunflower
and almond meal)

⅓ cup (45 g) sunflower seeds

⅓ cup (40 g) chopped walnuts

Preheat oven to 160°C (315°F)
fan-forced.

Beat eggs and oil together
until creamy. Stir in honey and
cinnamon until dissolved. Mix
in mashed bananas. Add flour
and LSA. Once mixed, add
sunflower seeds and walnuts
and stir until combined.

Grease a loaf tin (13 cm
× 24 cm) with oil and line the
base with baking paper.

Bake for 1 hour.

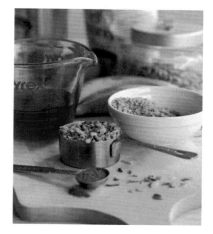

Check the centre of the cake with a skewer to make sure it is
cooked through; it may need another 5 minutes. Leave to cool
for 30 minutes in the tin. Run a blunt knife around the sides
of the cake to remove. Cool on a cake rack.

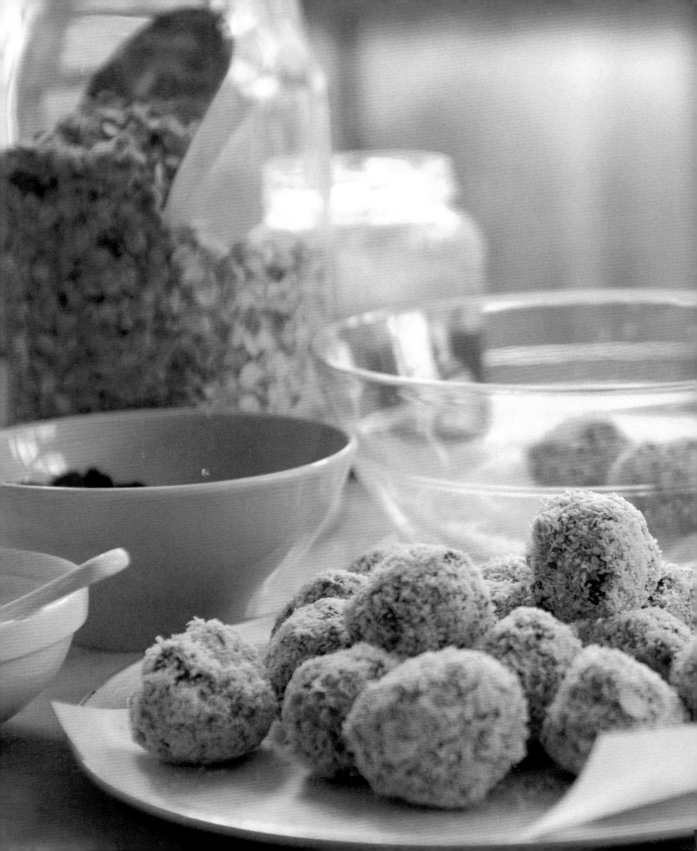

morning tea

When the tummy starts to rumble around 11 o'clock, a hot drink and a tempting treat will keep you going until lunchtime. Sometimes a piece of fruit or a handful of nuts just doesn't cut it. These delicious treats will satisfy your craving and are full of lots of healthy ingredients, so you won't feel guilty eating them! Now you can have your cake and eat it too.

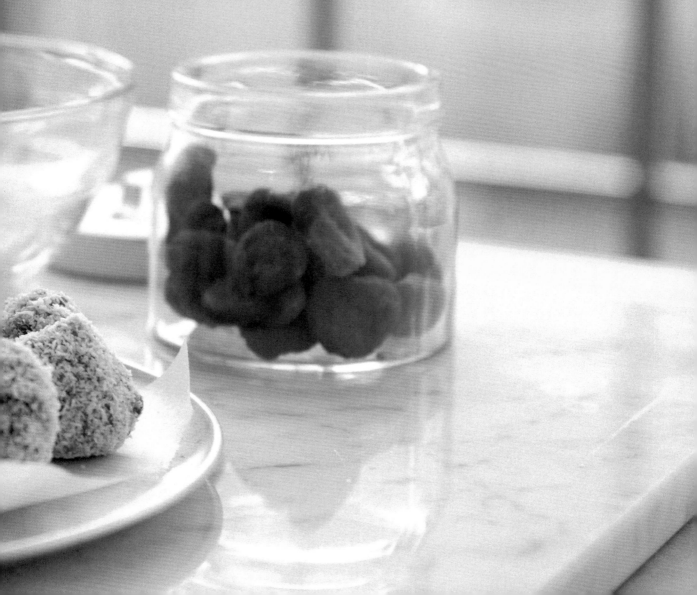

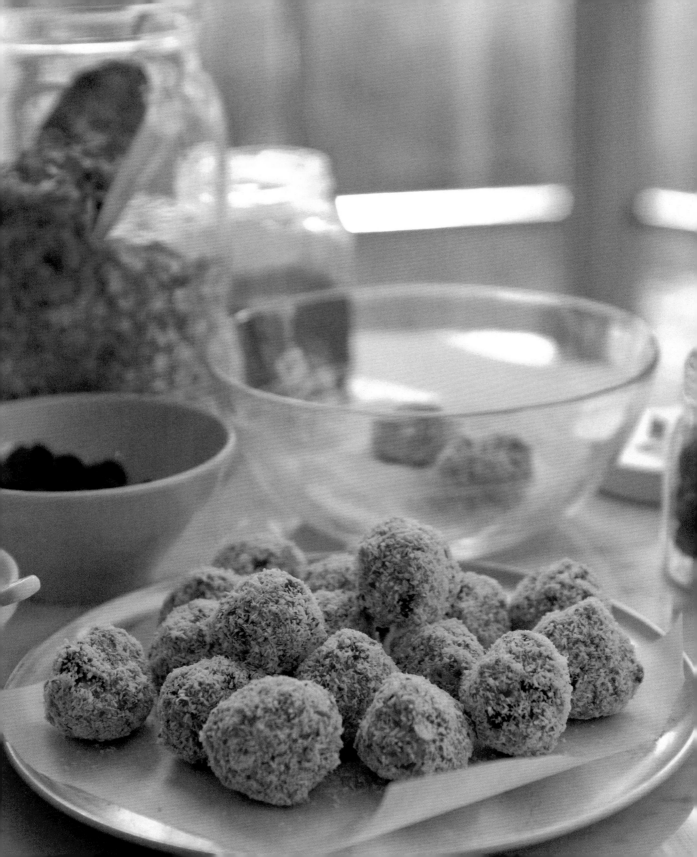

coconut muesli balls

ingredients

2 cups (210 g) toasted muesli
(see page 16)

1 cup (100 g) desiccated coconut,
plus extra to coat

½ cup (55 g) LSA (linseed, sunflower
and almond meal)

½ cup (150 g) honey

2 tablespoons boiled water

4 tablespoons hulled tahini

½ cup (70 g) organic dried apricots,
chopped

½ cup (70 g) sultanas

Mix toasted muesli, coconut and LSA in a bowl. Mix honey and water together until honey is dissolved. Stir honey mixture and tahini into the dry ingredients until thoroughly mixed through. Add apricots and sultanas.

Pour some extra coconut into a bowl. Firmly squeeze the mixture into small balls, then roll each one in coconut. Place them on a plate in the fridge. Once they are cold and firm, transfer them to an airtight container and return them to the fridge.

Makes 20 to 24.

apple and pecan muffins

ingredients

2 eggs

½ cup (125 ml) rice bran oil

½ cup (150 g) honey

1 teaspoon cinnamon

1¼ cups (280 g) cooked apples
(fresh or tinned)

½ cup (55 g) almond meal

1½ cups (240 g) wholemeal
(wholewheat) self-raising flour

⅔ cup (165 ml) milk

½ cup (55 g) chopped pecans

Preheat oven to 170°C (335°F) fan-forced.

Beat eggs and oil together. Mix in honey and cinnamon.

To cook apples, slice then place apples in a saucepan with some water. Bring to the boil, then reduce heat to low and simmer for 10 minutes. Drain apples. (If using tinned apples, make sure you buy a brand with no added sugar.)

Mash cooked apples gently with a fork and add to egg mixture.

Mix in almond meal, and then mix in flour and milk. Add the chopped pecans.

Grease muffin tins with oil and fill each case ¾ full. Place a whole pecan in the centre of each one.

Bake for 25 minutes.

Using a blunt knife, go around the edge of each one to help loosen them from the tin.

Makes 12.

apricot bread

ingredients

1 cup (145 g) organic dried apricots
1 cup (250 ml) boiling water
2 eggs
½ cup (125 ml) rice bran oil
¾ cup (225 g) honey
½ cup (50 g) desiccated coconut
2 cups (320 g) wholemeal
   (wholewheat) self-raising flour
½ cup (60 g) chopped walnuts

Preheat oven to 160°C (315°F) fan-forced.

Dice apricots, place in a bowl and cover with boiling water. Set aside to cool.

Beat eggs and oil together and mix in honey. Add coconut. Mix in flour and the water the apricots were soaked in, alternating between the two, until mixed in.

Use a spatula to press the apricots to extract all the water.

Mix in diced apricots and walnuts.

Grease a loaf tin (13 cm x 24 cm) with oil and line the base with baking paper. Pour in mixture.

Bake for 1 hour. Check with a skewer; it may need another 5 to 10 minutes, depending on your oven. Leave to cool in the tin for at least 20 minutes. Remove and leave to cool further on a cake rack.

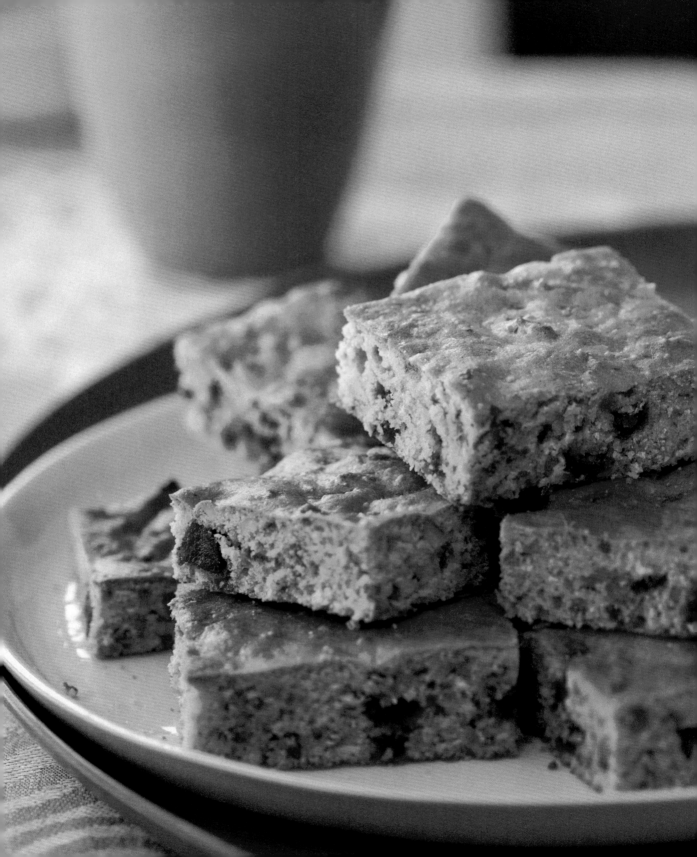

date and walnut slice

ingredients

3 eggs

⅓ cup (80 ml) rice bran oil

⅓ cup (95 g) honey

¾ cup (80 g) almond meal

½ cup (80 g) wholemeal
   (wholewheat) self-raising flour

¾ cup (105 g) chopped dates

½ cup (60 g) chopped walnuts

Preheat oven to 160°C (315°F) fan-forced.

Beat eggs, oil and honey together. Mix in almond meal and flour.

Cut dates into small pieces, separate them with your fingers and scatter over the top of the bowl before mixing them in as they can be quite sticky. This will ensure that they are spread evenly through the slice. Mix in chopped walnuts.

Grease a brownie tray (28 cm × 18 cm) with oil and line base with baking paper.

Bake for 25 minutes.

Leave to cool in the tin for 20 minutes. Remove and cool further on a cake rack.

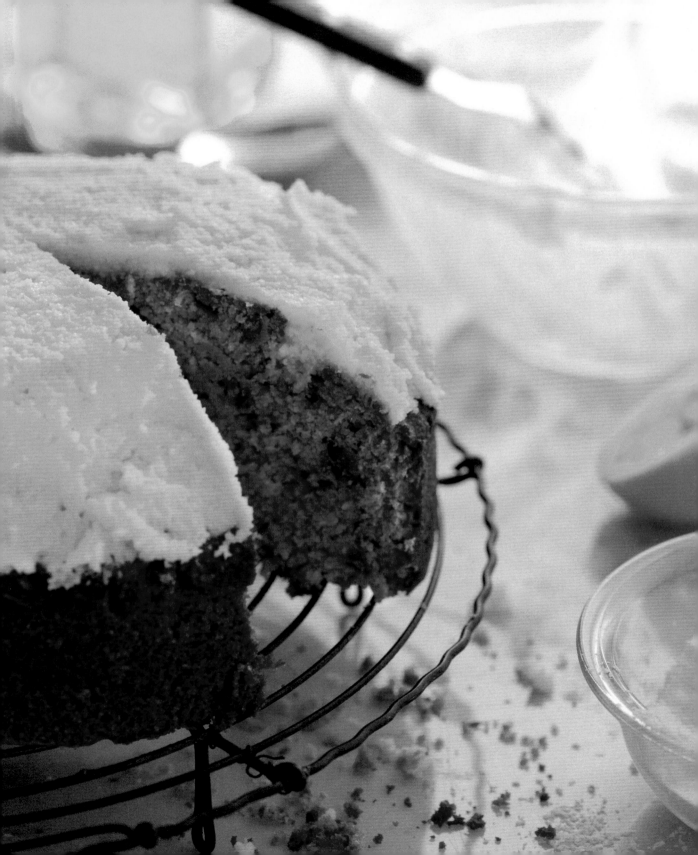

carrot cake

ingredients

cake

3 eggs

1 cup (250 ml) rice bran oil

¾ cup (225 g) honey

1½ teaspoons cinnamon

1½ cups (280 g) finely grated carrot

1 cup (100 g) desiccated coconut

2 cups (320 g) wholemeal
  (wholewheat) self-raising flour

¾ cup (80 g) chopped pecans

½ cup (70 g) sunflower seeds

icing

⅓ cup (75 g) ricotta

1½ tablespoons rice bran oil

¼ cup (75 g) honey

2 teaspoons lemon juice

¾ cup (75 g) desiccated coconut

Preheat oven to 160°C (315°F) fan-forced.

Beat eggs and oil together. Stir in honey and cinnamon. Grate carrot finely and press firmly into a measuring cup. Add carrot to mixture. Mix in coconut and flour and add chopped pecans and sunflower seeds.

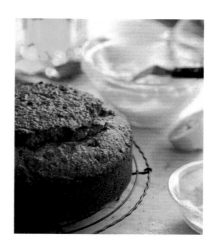

Grease a 20 cm round baking tin with oil and line the base with baking paper.

Bake for 1 hour. Check with a skewer; it may need 5 to 10 minutes more. Leave to cool in the tin for 20 minutes. Flip cake out and cool further on a cake rack.

To prepare icing, blend all ingredients together in a food processor. Spread icing over cake with a spatula.

Store in the refrigerator.

Hint: To save time, use a food processor to grate the carrot.

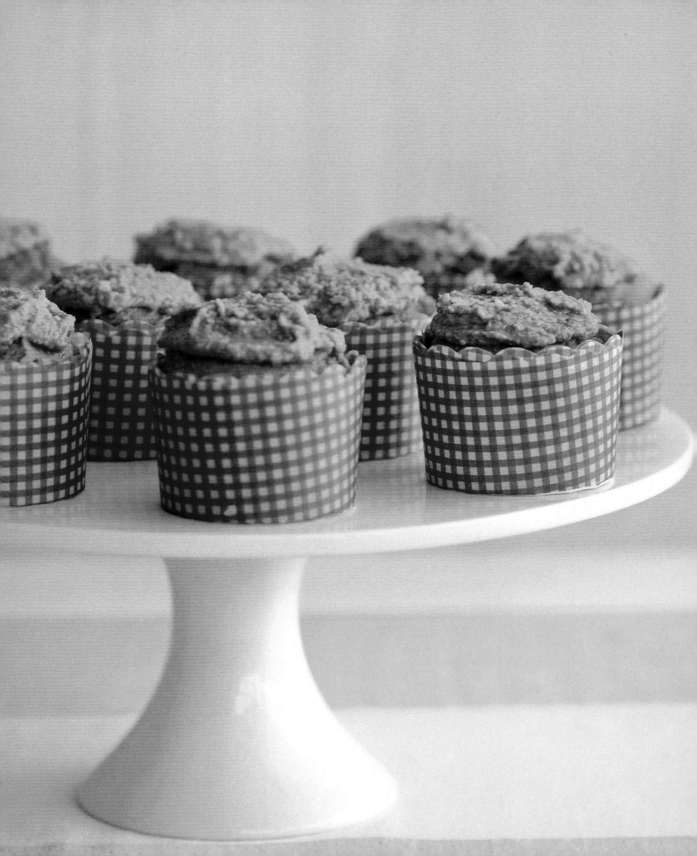

raspberry cupcakes

ingredients

cupcakes

2 eggs

½ cup (125 ml) rice bran oil

½ cup (150 g) honey

½ vanilla bean

1½ cups (240 g) wholemeal (wholewheat) self-raising flour

⅓ cup (80 ml) milk

1 cup (125 g) raspberries (fresh or frozen)

1 tablespoon boiling water

icing

¼ cup (60 g) ricotta

½ vanilla bean

2 tablespoons honey

1 teaspoon rice bran oil

½ cup (50 g) desiccated coconut

½ cup (65 g) raspberries (fresh or frozen)

Preheat oven to 170°C (335°F) fan-forced.

Beat eggs and oil together until creamy. Add honey and stir until dissolved. Slice vanilla bean lengthways and scrape out seeds from one half. Add seeds to mixture. Set aside the remaining half of the vanilla bean for the icing.

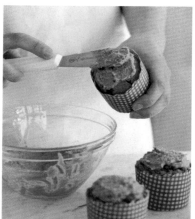

Mix in flour and milk. Blend raspberries and boiling water in a food processor until smooth and then add to the mixture.

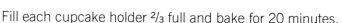

Fill each cupcake holder ⅔ full and bake for 20 minutes.

Once the cupcakes are cool, prepare the icing. Place ricotta, remaining vanilla bean seeds, honey, oil, coconut and raspberries in a food processor and blend until mixture is smooth. Cover each cupcake with icing and store in the refrigerator.

Makes 12.

Hint: Allow the raspberries to thaw a little before placing them in the food processor.

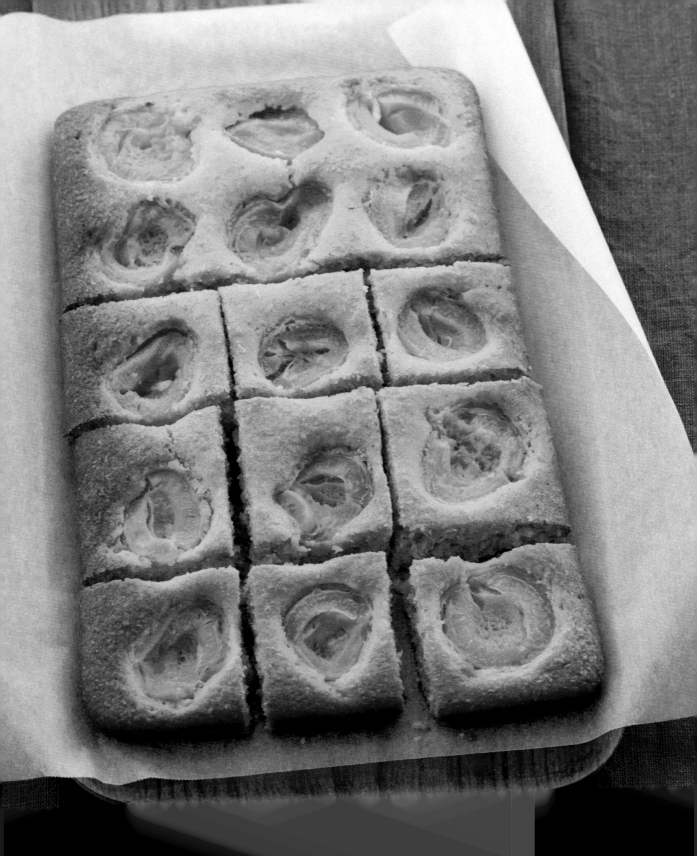

apricot slice

ingredients

3 eggs

⅓ cup (80 ml) rice bran oil

⅓ cup (95 g) honey

½ cup (50 g) desiccated coconut

¾ cup (120 g) wholemeal (wholewheat) self-raising flour

9 apricots, halved (fresh or tinned)

Preheat oven to 160°C (315°F) fan-forced.

Beat eggs, oil and honey together. Add coconut and flour and beat until mixed through.

Grease a brownie tray (28 cm × 18 cm) with oil and line the base with baking paper. Pour mixture into tin. Halve the apricots and place them evenly over the mixture, with the inside of the apricots facing up. If using tinned apricots, buy them with no added sugar and drain well.

Bake for 25 minutes.

Allow to cool and then slice.

flourless almond and coconut cake

ingredients

4 eggs

½ cup (125 ml) rice bran oil

½ cup (150 g) honey

¼ cup (60 ml) orange juice

1½ cups (165 g) almond meal

1 cup (100 g) desiccated coconut

1 tablespoon 100% apricot jam

2 tablespoons toasted almond flakes
   for decorating

Preheat oven to 160°C (315°F) fan-forced.

Separate eggs and beat egg whites until stiff. In a separate bowl beat together egg yolks, oil and honey. Add orange juice.

Mix almond meal and coconut into the egg yolk mixture until combined. Gently fold in egg whites.

Grease a 25 cm springform tin with oil and line the base with baking paper. Pour in mixture.

Bake for 35 to 40 minutes.

Leave cake to cool in the tin for at least 20 minutes. Remove and cool further on a cake rack.

Warm apricot jam in a saucepan on a low heat and then press it through a strainer to remove any lumps. Brush the jam over the cake and scatter toasted almond flakes around the edge of the cake (toast them first, for 8 minutes at 180°C (350°F) fan-forced).

passionfruit and citrus cake

ingredients

2 eggs

⅔ cup (165 ml) rice bran oil

½ cup (150 g) honey

½ teaspoon lemon rind

½ teaspoon orange rind

¼ cup (60 ml) orange juice

¼ cup (60 ml) passionfruit juice
   (3 to 4 passionfruits)

¾ cup (75 g) desiccated coconut

1 ½ cups (240 g) wholemeal
   (wholewheat) self-raising flour

1 tablespoon 100% apricot jam

desiccated coconut for decorating

Preheat oven to 160°C (315°F) fan-forced.

Beat eggs, oil and honey together. Finely grate lemon rind and orange rind and add to mixture (use the back of a spoon to rub the rind against the side of the bowl to make sure it dissolves into the mixture). Add orange juice.

Press the passionfruit pulp through a strainer to extract juice. Discard seeds and add juice to the mixture.

Mix in coconut and flour.

Grease an 18 cm square tin with oil and line the base with baking paper.

Bake for 40 minutes.

Leave cake to cool in the tin for at least 20 minutes. Remove and cool further on a cake rack.

When cake has cooled, warm apricot jam in a saucepan over a low heat and press through a strainer to remove any lumps. Brush top of cake with apricot jam and sprinkle with coconut.

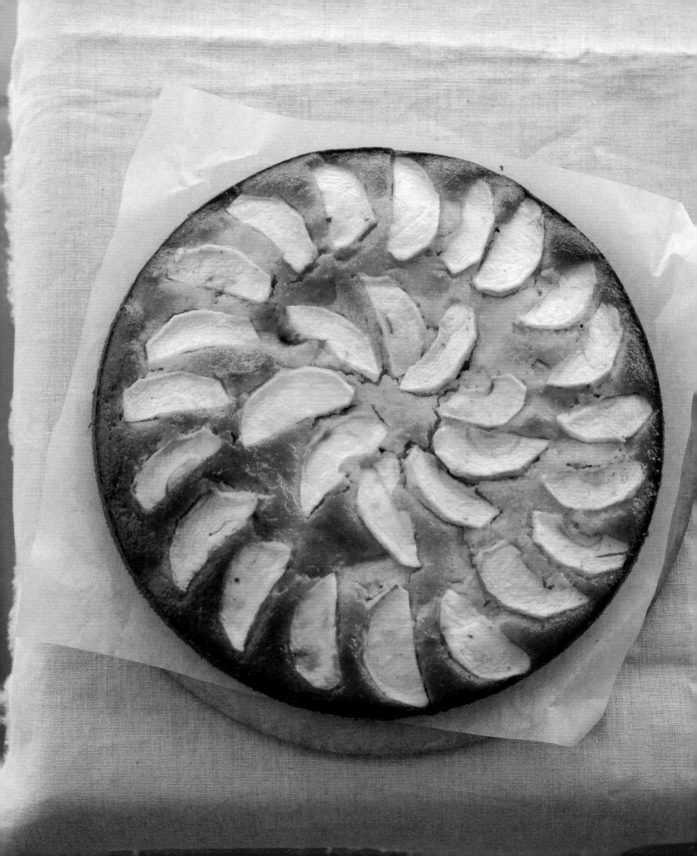

apple and almond cake

ingredients

2 eggs

½ cup (125 ml) rice bran oil

½ cup (150 g) honey

1½ cups (165 g) almond meal

¾ cup (120 g) wholemeal
  (wholewheat) self-raising flour

¼ cup (60 ml) milk

¼ cup (60 ml) boiling water

2 Granny Smith apples

2 tablespoons 100% apricot jam

Preheat the oven to 160°C (315°F) fan-forced.

Beat eggs and oil together until creamy. Add honey and mix until dissolved. Mix in almond meal and then flour. Add milk. Add boiling water and beat until all ingredients are mixed through.

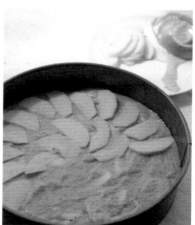

Peel the apples. Slice into quarters, remove cores, and cut each quarter into thin slices. Fold approximately one and a half apples into the mixture, leaving enough slices to decorate the top of the cake.

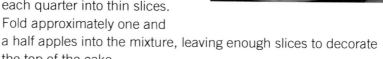

Grease a 25 cm springform tin with oil and line the base with baking paper. Pour mixture into tin and decorate with remaining apple slices.

Bake for 40 minutes. Check the centre of the cake with a skewer to ensure that it is cooked through.

Place jam in a saucepan and warm on a low heat. Press through a strainer so you have a smooth jam. Brush jam over the apple cake.

Allow cake to cool in tin for 20 to 30 minutes. Remove from tin and cool futher on a cake rack.

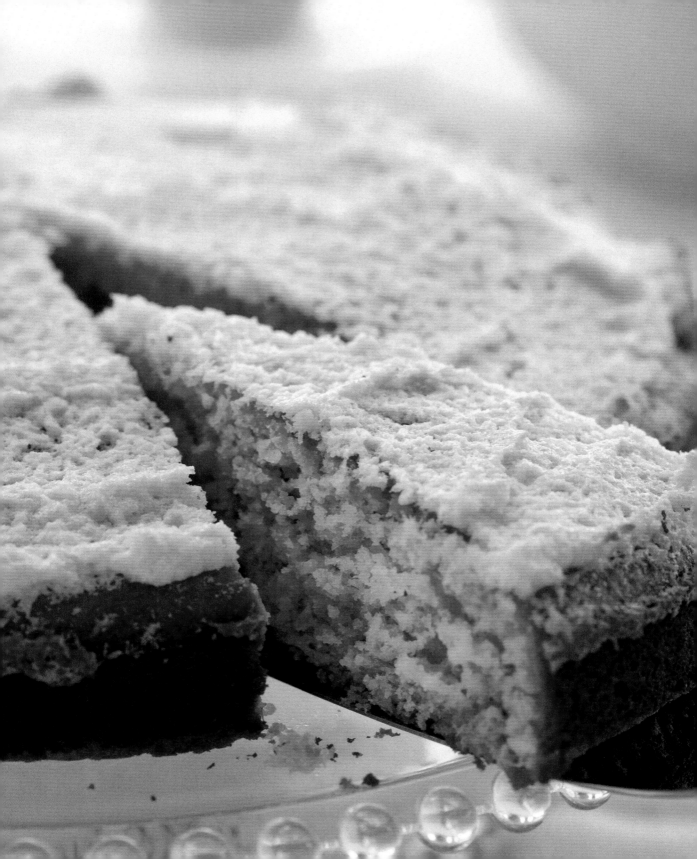

lemon and coconut meringue cake

ingredients

cake

2 eggs

1 egg yolk

½ cup (125 ml) rice bran oil

½ cup (150 g) honey

½ cup (55 g) almond meal

½ cup (50 g) desiccated coconut

75 ml lemon juice

1½ cups (240 g) wholemeal
   (wholewheat) self-raising flour

½ cup (125 ml) milk

topping

2 egg whites

1 tablespoon honey

½ cup (50 g) desiccated coconut

Preheat oven to 160°C (315°F) fan-forced.

Beat eggs, egg yolk and oil together. Add honey. Mix in almond meal and coconut. Add lemon juice and mix in flour and milk.

Grease a 25 cm springform tin with oil and line the base with baking paper.

Bake for 30 minutes.

To prepare topping, beat egg whites together with honey until stiff. Gently fold in coconut until mixed through.

When the cake has baked for 30 minutes remove from oven and using a spatula cover the top of the cake with the meringue mix. Bake for a further 10 minutes.

Leave cake in tin until it has cooled as this makes it easier to remove. Run a knife around the edge of the cake to help loosen it. After removing the outside of the tin, gently place your hand over the top of the cake to remove the base and leave it to cool further on a cake rack.

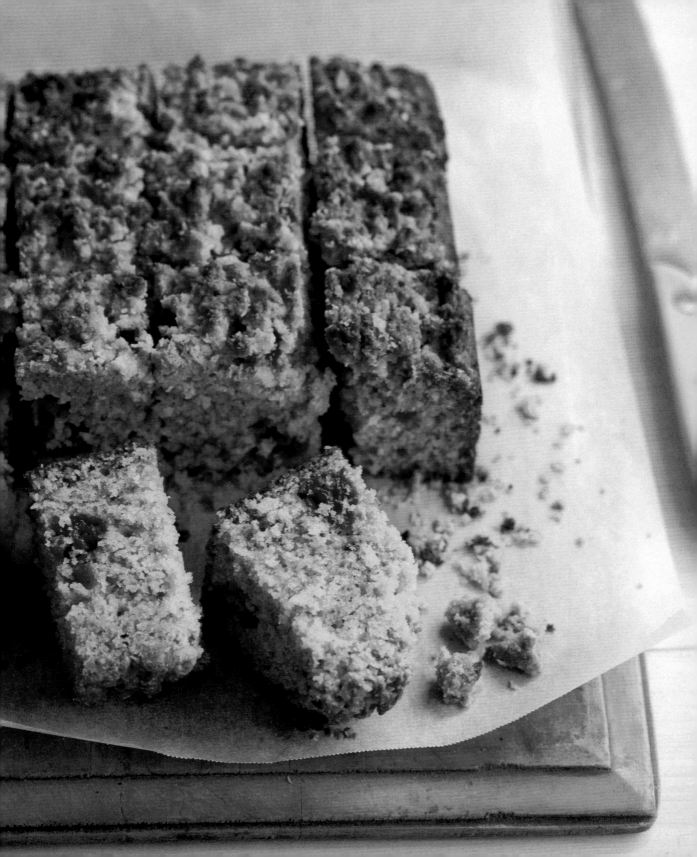

raspberry and orange cake with coconut crumble

ingredients

cake

2 eggs

¾ cup (185 ml) rice bran oil

¾ cup (225 g) honey

1 teaspoon finely grated orange rind

½ cup (55 g) almond meal

¼ cup (25 g) desiccated coconut

1¾ cups (280 g) wholemeal (wholewheat) self-raising flour

½ cup (125 ml) orange juice

1½ cups (190 g) raspberries (fresh or frozen)

crumble

⅓ cup (55 g) wholemeal (wholewheat) plain flour

⅓ cup (30 g) desiccated coconut

¼ cup (60 ml) rice bran oil

1½ tablespoons honey

Preheat oven to 160°C (315°F) fan-forced.

Beat eggs and oil together. Stir in honey and orange rind. Add almond meal and coconut and mix in flour and orange juice.

Grease an 18 cm square tin with oil and line the base with baking paper. Pour mixture into tin and place half the raspberries evenly over the top. Gently push each one into the mixture. Place the remaining raspberries evenly over the top of the mixture.

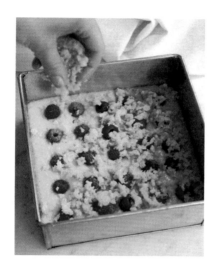

To prepare crumble, mix flour and coconut together in a bowl. In a separate bowl, mix oil and honey together, then mix in the dry ingredients. Scatter crumble evenly over cake.

Bake for 1 hour 10 minutes to 1 hour 15 minutes (check with a skewer to make sure it has cooked through). Cool in tin for at least 20 minutes. Remove and cool further on a cake rack.

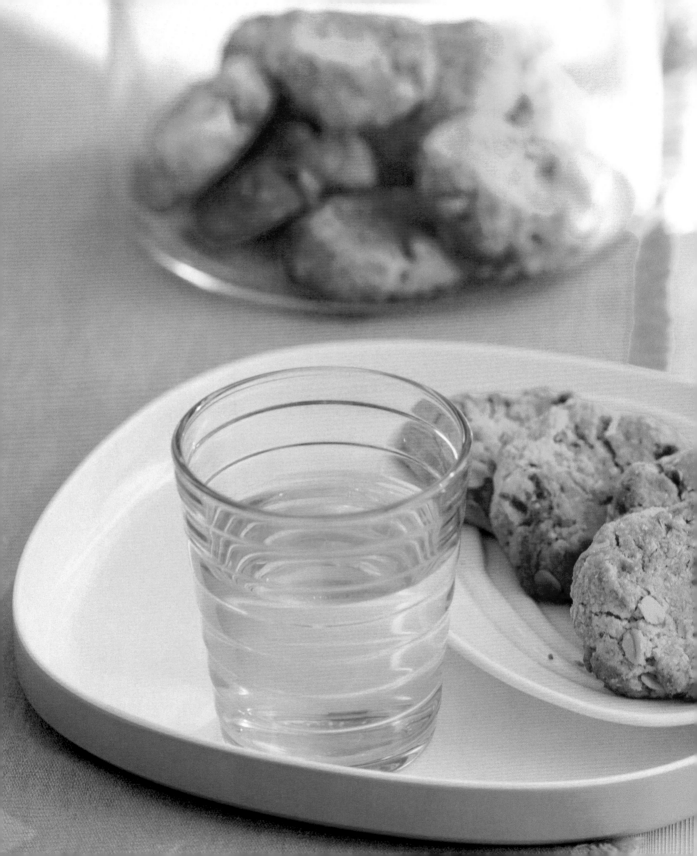

lunchbox treats

Now you can send your kids to school with a tasty nut-free treat full of healthy ingredients (they're also great to take to work). Your children will be happy because they have a cookie or muffin that looks and tastes like a 'normal' cookie or muffin and as parents we are comforted by the fact that these treats are full of fibre, low in sugars and low in saturated fat, without lots of preservatives or additives, and will give them the energy they need throughout their day.

I like to freeze muffins or cake slices individually. That way I can take them out of the freezer the night before and the kids can have something different in their lunches every day – a great option for working parents.

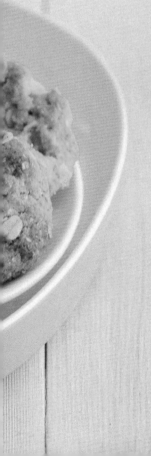

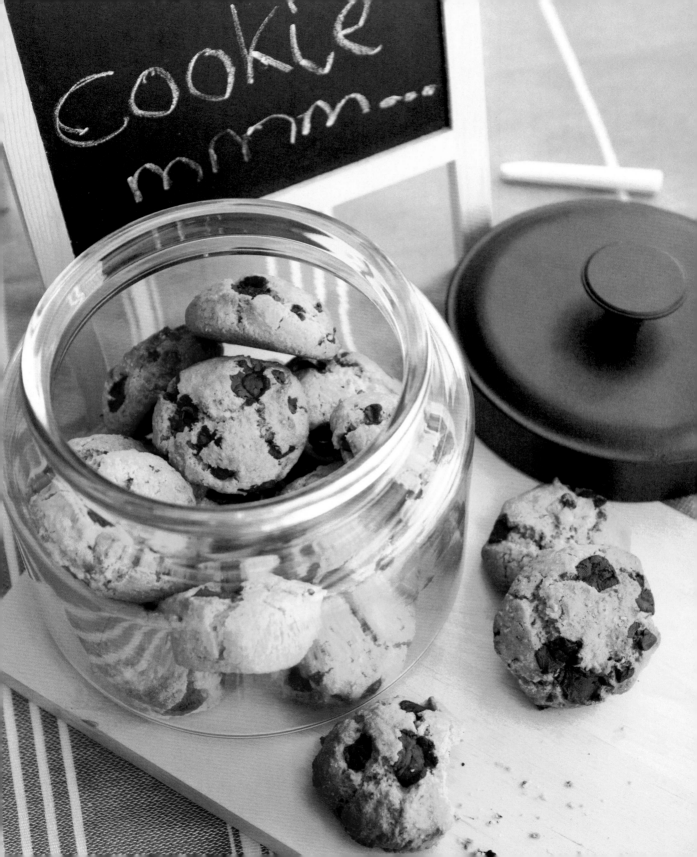

chocolate chip cookies

ingredients

1 egg

½ cup (125 ml) rice bran oil

½ cup (150 g) honey

¼ cup (60 ml) water

¼ cup (25 g) desiccated coconut

2 cups (320 g) wholemeal (wholewheat) self-raising flour

⅔ cup (90 g) chopped 70% dark chocolate

Preheat oven to 180°C (350°F) fan-forced.

Mix egg and oil together. Dissolve honey with water and add to egg mixture. Stir in coconut and flour and then add chocolate.

Leave mixture to stand for 10 minutes. This will make the mixture less sticky when rolling into balls. If you don't have time to let the mixture stand, use 2 teaspoons to spoon the mixture into dollops on the tray.

Line 2 trays with baking paper and place the balls on the trays.

Bake for 15 minutes.

Leave to cool for 5 minutes before placing cookies on a cake rack.

Makes 20 to 24.

Hint: I usually swap the position of the trays after 13 minutes as ovens often cook unevenly.

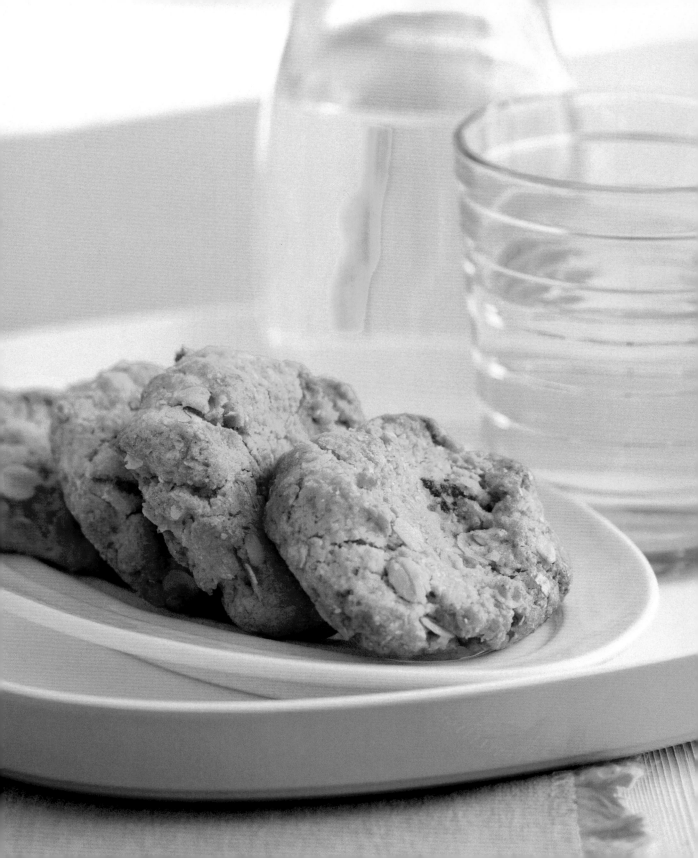

orange and fig biscuits

ingredients

1 cup (160 g) wholemeal
(wholewheat) self-raising flour

⅓ cup (30 g) desiccated coconut

⅓ cup (30 g) rolled oats

½ cup (125 ml) rice bran oil

⅓ cup (95 g) honey

½ teaspoon finely grated orange rind

2 tablespoons orange juice

⅓ cup (55 g) chopped dried figs

Preheat oven to 170°C (335°F) fan-forced.

Mix flour, coconut and oats together. In a separate bowl mix together oil, honey, orange rind and orange juice, then stir the mixture into the dry ingredients. Add chopped figs.

Leave to stand for 10 minutes then roll into balls. Press your thumb gently into the centre of each ball.

Bake for 15 minutes.

Makes 16.

coconut macaroons

ingredients

2 egg whites

¼ cup (75 g) honey

1½ cups (150 g) desiccated coconut

Preheat oven to 150°C (300°F) fan-forced.

Beat egg whites until stiff, add honey and beat until mixed through. Gently fold coconut into egg white mixture. Roll into small balls and place on a tray lined with baking paper.

Bake for 15 minutes at 150°C (300°F), reduce the temperature to 110°C (230°F) (don't remove from the oven) and bake for a further 15 minutes or until golden.

Makes 8 to 10.

sultana and sunflower cookies

ingredients

1 egg

½ cup (125 ml) rice bran oil

⅓ cup (95 g) honey

½ cup (50 g) desiccated coconut

1½ cups (240 g) wholemeal
   (wholewheat) self-raising flour

2 tablespoons water

¾ cup (105 g) sultanas

⅓ cup (45 g) sunflower seeds

Preheat oven to 180°C (350°F) fan-forced.

Mix egg, oil and honey together. Add coconut and flour and mix through. Add water.

Mix in sultanas and sunflower seeds.

Line 2 baking trays with baking paper. Shape mixture into small balls and flatten slightly with the palm of your hand.

Bake for 12 minutes or until golden (the bottom tray may need an extra 2 minutes).

Makes 24.

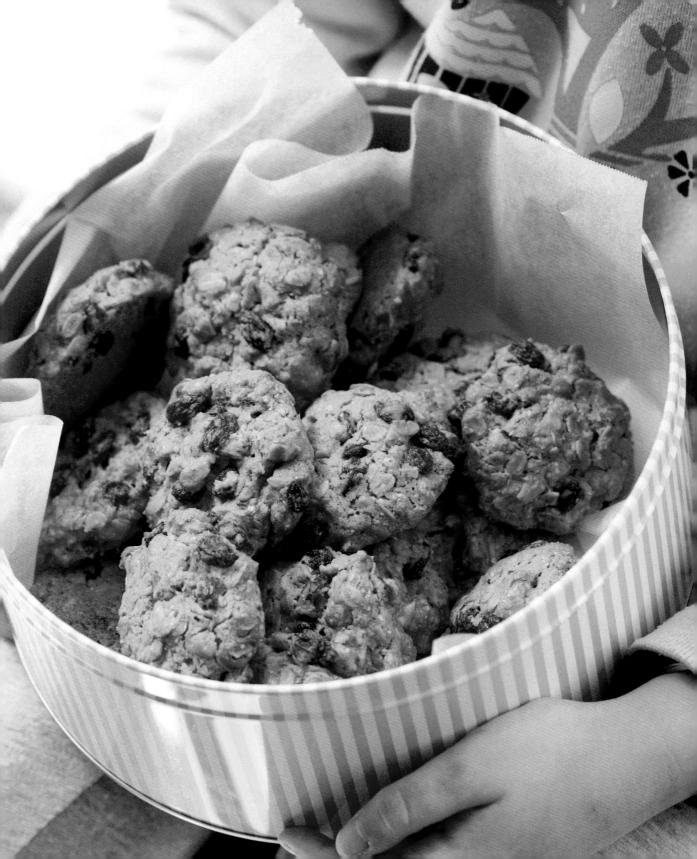

muesli biscuits

ingredients

2 cups (210 g) toasted muesli
(see page 16)

1 cup (160 g) wholemeal
(wholewheat) plain flour

½ cup (70 g) sultanas

1 teaspoon bi-carb soda

2 tablespoons boiled water

½ cup (150 g) honey

½ cup (125 ml) rice bran oil

Preheat oven to 150°C (300°F) fan-forced.

Mix toasted muesli, flour and sultanas in a bowl. In another bowl dissolve bi-carb soda in water and add honey and oil, stir until the mixture is smooth. Stir honey mixture into the dry ingredients.

Line 2 trays with baking paper. Shape into balls and place onto tray.

Bake for 15 minutes.

Makes 16 to 20.

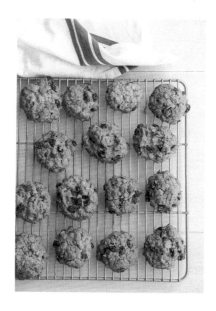

Hint: If you leave the mixture to stand for 15 to 20 minutes it's less sticky and easier to roll into balls.

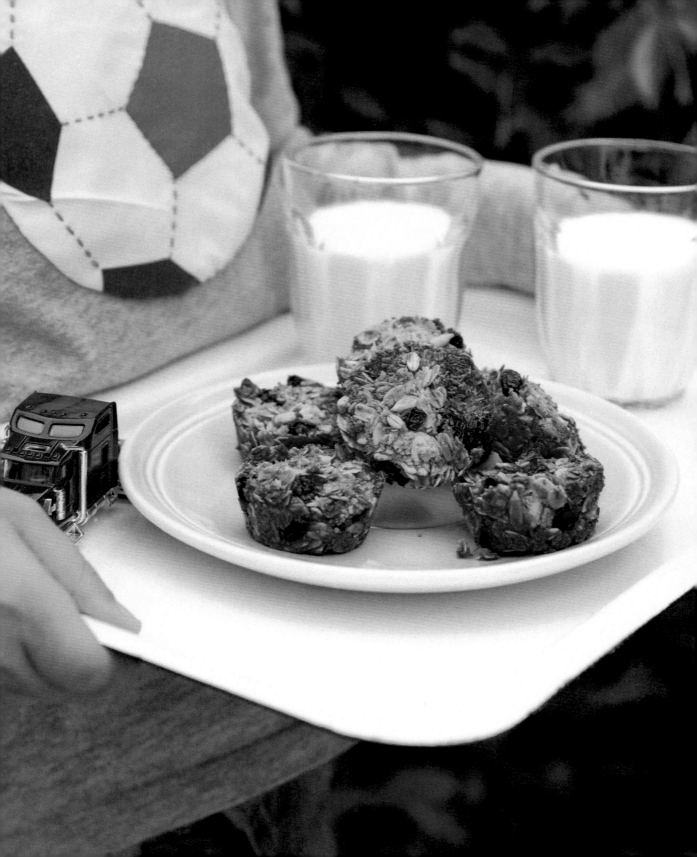

apricot muesli bites

ingredients

1¼ cups (125 g) rolled oats

1 cup (100 g) desiccated coconut

½ teaspoon cinnamon

½ cup (70 g) sunflower seeds

½ cup (70 g) sultanas

½ cup (70 g) organic dried apricots

½ cup (150 g) honey

⅓ cup (80 ml) rice bran oil

1 tablespoon boiling water

1 egg white

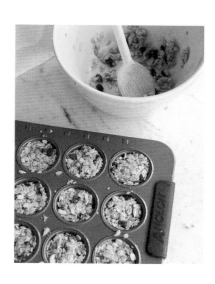

Preheat oven to 170°C (335°F) fan-forced.

Mix rolled oats, coconut, cinnamon, sunflower seeds and sultanas in a bowl. Cut apricots into small pieces and add to dry ingredients.

In a separate bowl, mix honey, oil and water until honey is dissolved. Mix into the dry ingredients. Add egg white and mix thoroughly.

Grease a mini muffin tin well with oil and fill each case with mixture. Using the back of a spoon or your fingers press mixture firmly in.

Bake for 25 minutes.

Leave to cool completely in the muffin tin.

Use a knife to go around the edges of each one to help lift them out.

Store in the fridge.

Makes 24.

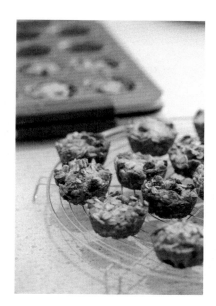

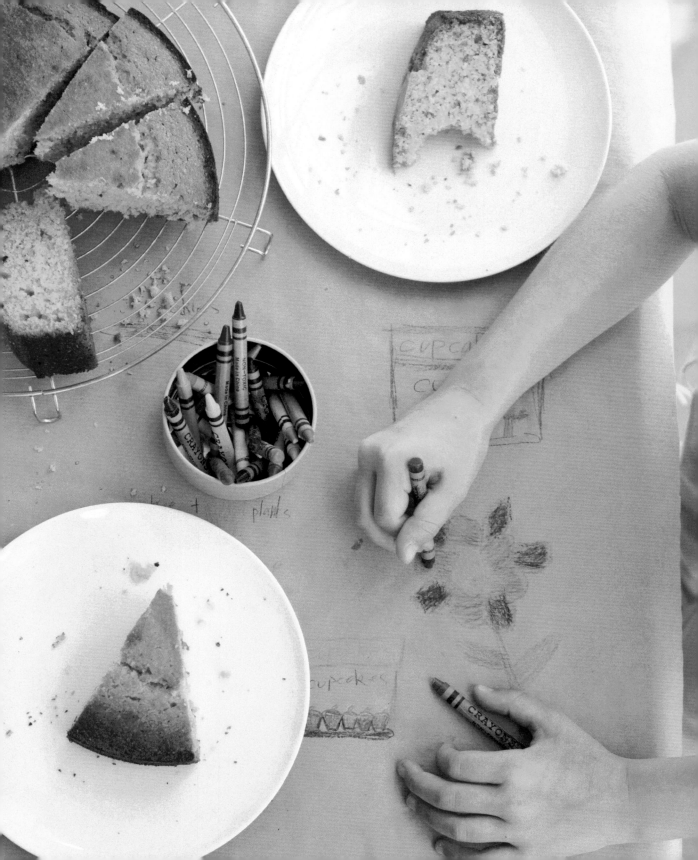

butterless butter cake

ingredients

2 eggs

1 egg yolk

¾ cup (185 ml) rice bran oil

½ cup (150 g) honey

½ cup (125 ml) orange juice

1 vanilla bean

⅓ cup (30 g) desiccated coconut

1½ cups (240 g) wholemeal
   (wholewheat) self-raising flour

Preheat oven to 160°C (315°F) fan-forced.

Beat eggs, egg yolk and oil together until creamy. Stir in honey until dissolved. Add orange juice.

Cut vanilla bean lengthways and scrape out seeds. Add vanilla bean seeds to mixture; use the back of a spoon to rub seeds against the side of the bowl to ensure they dissolve into the mixture. Mix in coconut and flour.

Grease a 20 cm round tin with oil and line base with baking paper. Pour in mixture.

Bake for 40 minutes.

Leave to cool in tin for 20 minutes. Remove and leave to cool further on a cake rack.

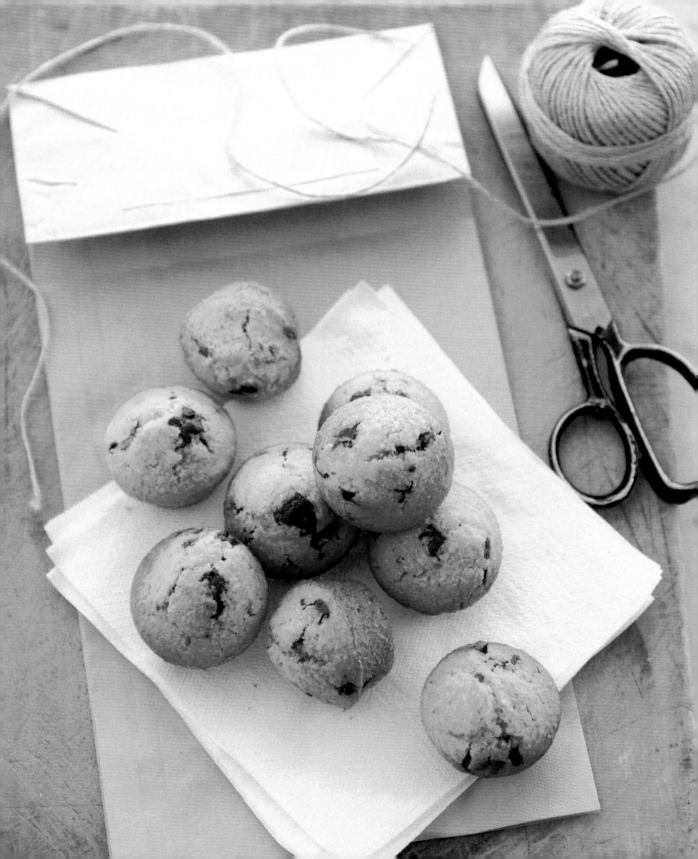

mini choc chip muffins

ingredients

1 egg

¼ cup (60 ml) rice bran oil

¼ cup (75 g) honey

¾ cup (120 g) wholemeal (wholewheat) self-raising flour

¼ cup (25 g) desiccated coconut

⅓ cup (80 ml) milk

⅓ cup (45 g) chopped 70% dark chocolate

Preheat oven to 180°C (350°F) fan-forced.

Whisk egg, oil and honey together until honey is dissolved. Mix in flour, coconut and milk then add chocolate.

Grease mini muffin tin with oil and fill each case ¾ full.

Bake for 15 minutes.

Makes 12.

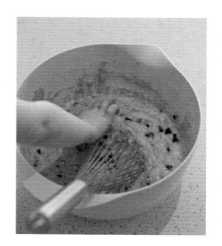 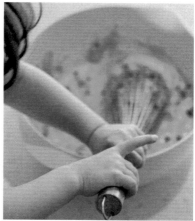 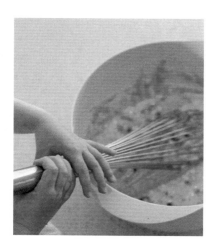

banana muffins

ingredients

2 eggs

½ cup (125 ml) rice bran oil

½ cup (150 g) honey

3 bananas, mashed

1 teaspoon cinnamon

½ cup (50 g) desiccated coconut

2 cups (320 g) wholemeal (wholewheat) self-raising flour

½ cup (125 ml) milk

½ cup (65 g) chopped 70% dark chocolate

Preheat oven to 170°C (335°F) fan-forced.

Beat eggs, oil and honey together. Add mashed banana and cinnamon. Mix in coconut, flour and milk, then mix in chopped dark chocolate.

Grease a muffin tin with oil (or you can use muffin holders). Fill each case ¾ full.

Bake for 20 minutes.

Leave to cool in tin, then go around each muffin, carefully, with a blunt knife to make sure they are not stuck to the sides before removing them.

Makes 12.

chocolate and raspberry muffins

ingredients

2 eggs

½ cup (125 ml) rice bran oil

100 g 70% dark chocolate

½ cup (150 g) honey

¼ cup (25 g) desiccated coconut

1½ cups (240 g) wholemeal
(wholewheat) self-raising flour

¾ cup (185 ml) milk

1 cup (125 g) raspberries (fresh or
frozen)

Preheat oven to 170°C (335°F) fan-forced.

Beat eggs and oil together.

Melt chocolate and stir honey into chocolate until dissolved. Pour chocolate mixture into egg mix and add coconut, flour and milk.

Once ingredients are mixed through, fold in the raspberries using a spatula.

Grease a muffin tin with oil and fill each case ¾ full.

Bake for 20 minutes. Leave to cool in the muffin tin for at least 10 minutes before removing and cooling on a cake rack.

Makes 12.

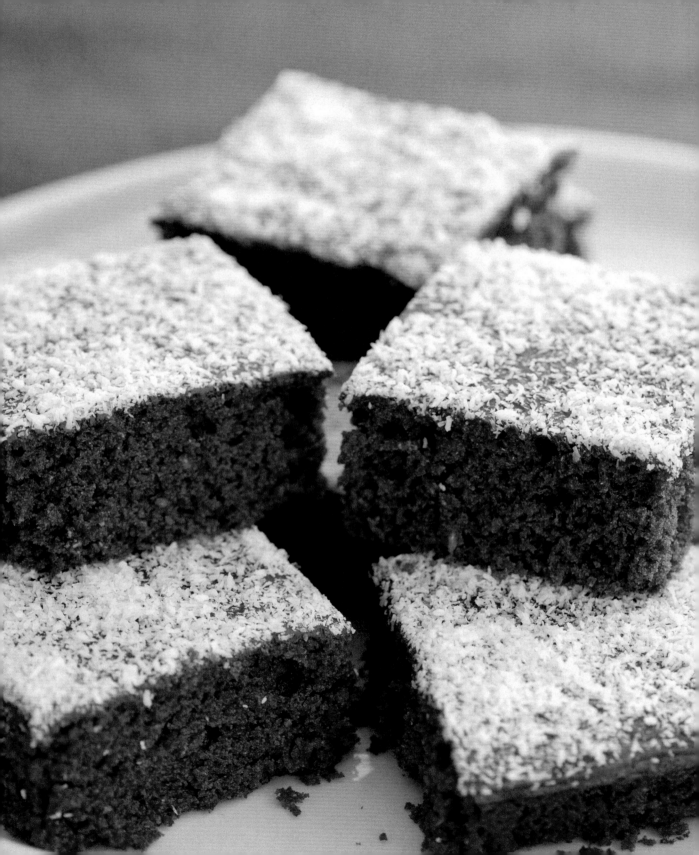

afternoon tea

Afternoon tea is the time of day when you need a snack to keep going until dinner. This section has lots of delicious cakes and treats, full of healthy ingredients, for a Sunday afternoon or when entertaining guests. Get cosy by the fire and have some scones with jam, a dreamy cake or tart, or a heavenly friand.

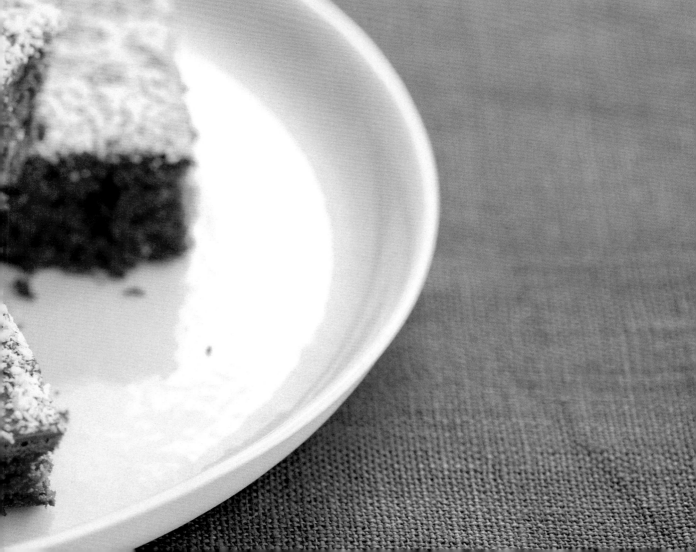

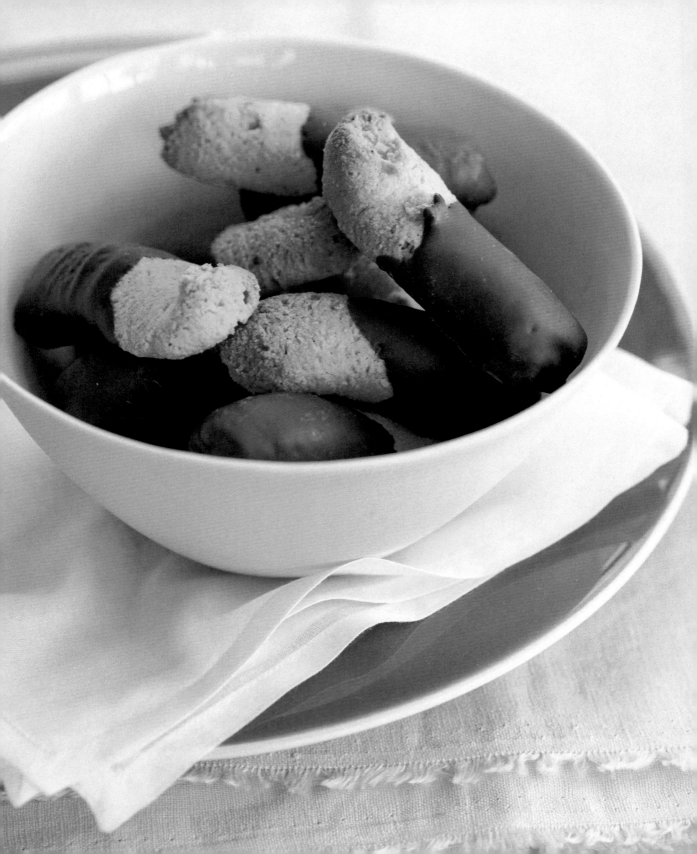

almond and chocolate biscuits

ingredients

3 egg whites

¾ cup (225 g) honey

3 cups (330 g) almond meal

¼ cup (40 g) wholemeal (wholewheat) plain flour

150 g 70% dark chocolate

Preheat oven to 140°C (285°F) fan-forced.

Beat egg whites until stiff. Add honey and beat until mixed through.

In a separate bowl mix together almond meal and flour. Gently fold dry ingredients into the egg whites.

Line 2 trays with baking paper. Use a piping bag to pipe the mixture onto trays in the shape of sticks, roughly 7.5 cm in length.

Bake for 30 minutes.

Leave to cool for 5 to 10 minutes before placing biscuits on a cake rack.

Once cooled, melt dark chocolate and coat each biscuit, covering ²/₃ with chocolate.

Place biscuits on a tray with foil and refrigerate to set. When the chocolate has set, store the biscuits in a container in the fridge.

Makes 32.

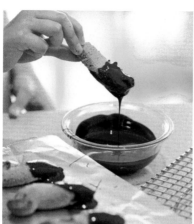

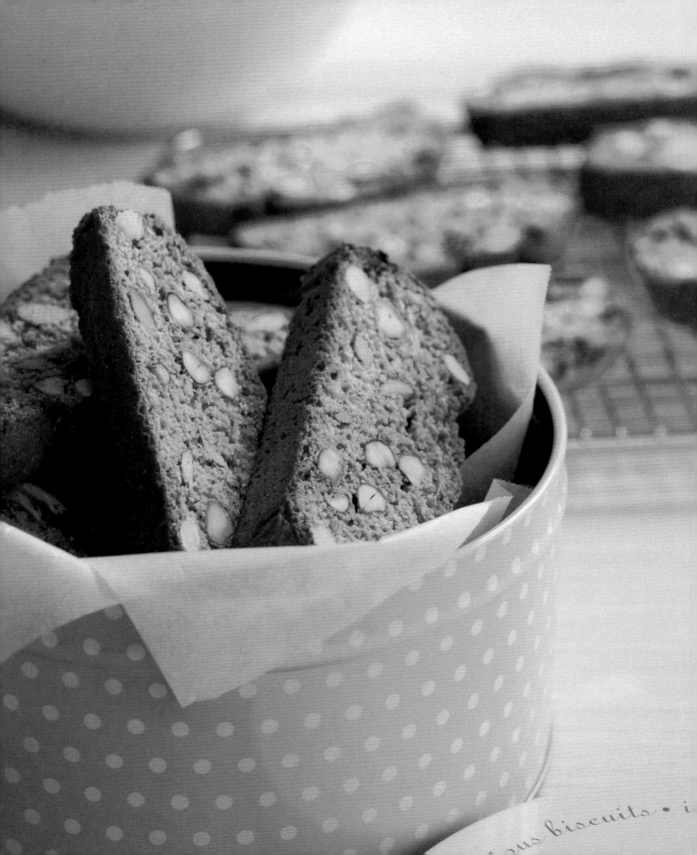

honey, pistachio and almond biscotti

ingredients

3 eggs

¾ cup (225 g) honey

1 teaspoon finely grated orange rind

1 vanilla bean

3 tablespoons desiccated coconut

2¼ cups (360 g) wholemeal (wholewheat) self-raising flour

⅔ cup (85 g) chopped almonds

⅔ cup (75 g) pistachios

½ cup (65 g) chopped 70% dark chocolate

Preheat oven to 160°C (315°F) fan-forced.

Beat eggs, honey, orange rind and vanilla bean seeds in a bowl (to extract seeds cut vanilla bean lengthways and scrape out seeds). Use a spoon to mix in coconut and flour. Once mixed through, stir in chopped almonds, pistachios and chocolate.

Line a tray with baking paper, make 3 logs from the mixture and place on a tray.

Bake for 30 minutes.

Leave logs to cool on a rack. Once cooled, carefully slice them roughly 1 cm thick, and return to tray. Bake for 10 minutes. Turn each piece over and bake for another 10 minutes.

Place on a cake rack to cool.

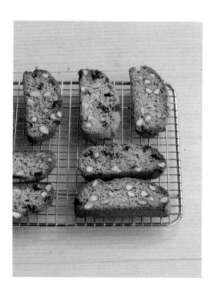

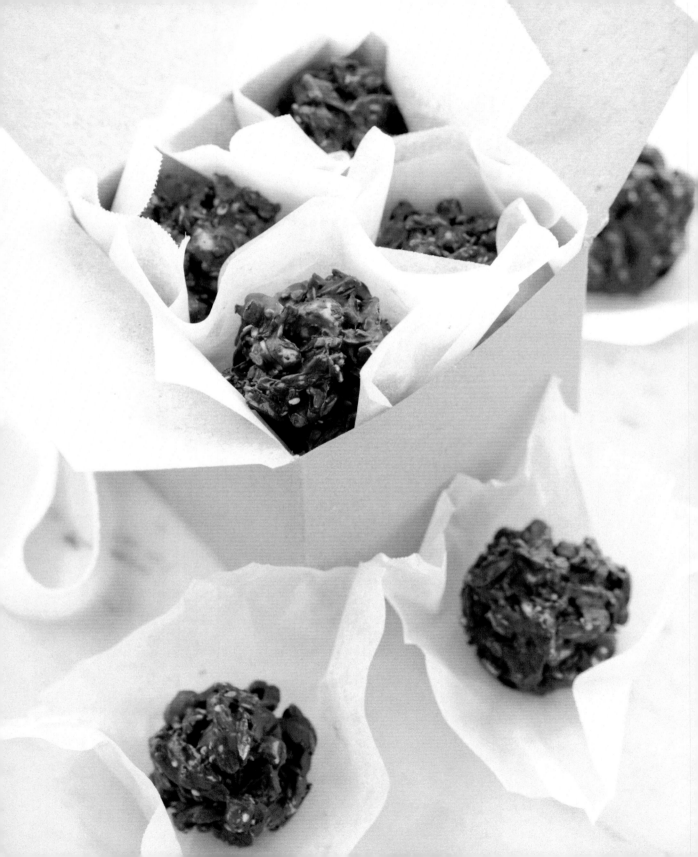

chocolate nut clusters

ingredients

½ cup (60 g) toasted slivered
   almonds

½ cup (65 g) chopped hazelnuts

⅓ cup (45 g) sunflower seeds

1 tablespoon sesame seeds

120 g 70% dark chocolate

2 tablespoons honey

Preheat oven to 180°C (350°F)
fan-forced.

Toast slivered almonds in oven
for 8 to 10 minutes, then set
aside to cool.

Place toasted almonds,
chopped hazelnuts, sunflower
seeds and sesame seeds in a
bowl and mix.

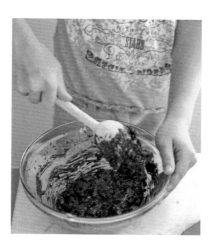

Melt dark chocolate. Stir in
honey until mixed through.

Combine chocolate mixture
with nut mixture until all the nuts are coated with chocolate.

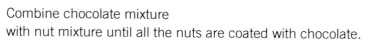

Lightly grease a mini muffin tin with oil and use a teaspoon to
place dollops of mixture into each case. Refrigerate for at least
2 hours before serving.

Store in an airtight container in the fridge.

Makes 12.

jam button biscuits

ingredients

1 egg

½ cup (125 ml) rice bran oil

⅓ cup (95 g) honey

½ teaspoon finely grated orange rind

1 cup (160 g) wholemeal
(wholewheat) plain flour

¾ cup (80 g) almond meal

⅓ cup (95 g) 100% strawberry jam

Preheat oven to 160°C (315°F) fan-forced.

Whisk egg, oil and honey together. Stir in orange rind. Use the back of a spoon to rub rind against the side of the bowl to make sure it dissolves into the mixture.

Whisk in flour and almond meal.

Warm strawberry jam in a saucepan over a low heat and then pour into a strainer. Press through with a teaspoon so you are left with a smooth jam.

Line 2 baking trays with baking paper. Roll mixture into small balls and make a hole in the centre with your index finger. Make sure you don't go through to the other side. Use a teaspoon to fill the centre of each biscuit with a dollop of jam.

Bake for 15 to 18 minutes.

Allow to cool on a cake rack.

Makes 20.

chocolate madeleines

ingredients

3 eggs

½ cup (125 ml) rice bran oil

80 g 70% dark chocolate

⅓ cup (95 g) honey

⅔ cup (110 g) wholemeal
   (wholewheat) self-raising flour

Preheat oven to 170°C (335°F) fan-forced.

Beat eggs and oil together until creamy. Melt chocolate. Add honey to chocolate and stir until dissolved. Mix into egg mixture.

Mix in flour and refrigerate for 15 minutes.

Grease a madeleine tin with oil and fill each case with mixture.

Bake for 13 to 15 minutes or until madeleines feel springy to touch.

Allow to cool in tin before lifting out.

Makes 24.

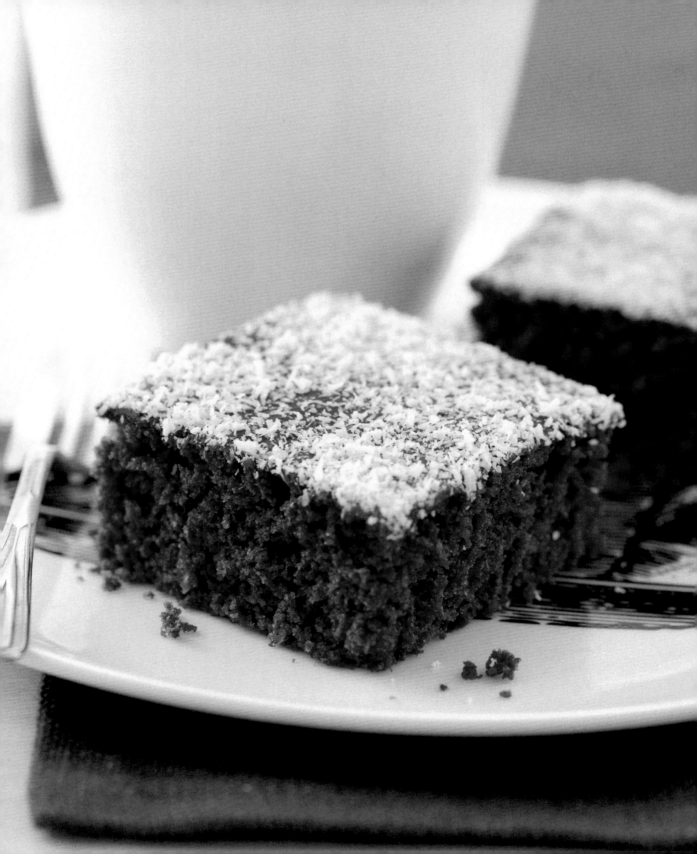

chocolate coconut slice

ingredients

slice

2 eggs, separated

½ cup (125 ml) rice bran oil

120 g 70% dark chocolate

½ cup (150 g) honey

½ cup (80 g) wholemeal
  (wholewheat) self-raising flour

½ cup (50 g) desiccated coconut

icing

50 g 70% dark chocolate

1 tablespoon honey

desiccated coconut for decoration

Preheat oven to 160°C (315°F) fan-forced.

Beat egg whites until stiff.

In a separate bowl beat egg yolks and oil. Melt chocolate and stir in honey until dissolved. Add chocolate mixture to the egg yolks and oil. Mix in flour and coconut and stir until combined.

Use a spatula to gently fold egg whites into chocolate mixture.

Grease a brownie tray (28 cm × 18 cm) with oil and line the base with baking paper.

Bake for 25 minutes.

Leave to cool in tin for 20 minutes before turning out onto a cake rack.

Once slice is cool, prepare the icing. Melt chocolate and stir in honey. Spread icing over the slice and sprinkle with coconut.

orange cake

ingredients

2 eggs

⅔ cup (165 ml) rice bran oil

⅔ cup (190 g) honey

2½ teaspoons finely grated orange rind

¾ cup (80 g) almond meal

1½ cups (240 g) wholemeal (wholewheat) self-raising flour

⅔ cup (165 ml) orange juice

Preheat oven to 160°C (315°F) fan-forced.

Beat eggs and oil together and dissolve honey into mixture. Stir in orange rind (use the back of a spoon to rub rind against side of bowl to make sure it properly dissolves in the mixture). Mix in almond meal, then flour and orange juice.

Line a 20 cm round tin with baking paper and grease sides with oil.

Bake for 50 minutes. Check centre of cake with a skewer to make sure it is cooked through.

Allow to cool in the tin for at least 20 minutes before removing and cooling on a cake rack.

Hint: For a more gourmet look, once the cake has cooled, brush with 100% apricot jam and sprinkle with toasted almond flakes. To prepare apricot jam, place 1 tablespoon of jam in a saucepan, on a low heat, and press through a strainer to remove any lumps.

coconut cupcakes

ingredients

cupcakes

2 eggs

½ cup (125 ml) rice bran oil

½ cup (150 g) honey

1 cup (100 g) desiccated coconut

1½ cups (240 g) wholemeal
   (wholewheat) self-raising flour

½ cup (125 ml) milk

icing

¼ cup (60 g) ricotta

2 tablespoons honey

1 teaspoon rice bran oil

½ cup (50 g) desiccated coconut

1 tablespoon orange juice

Preheat oven to 170°C (335°F) fan-forced.

Beat eggs, oil and honey together. Add coconut and stir. Mix in flour and milk.

Pour mixture into cupcake holders, filling ⅔ full and bake for 18 minutes.

To prepare icing place all ingredients in a food processor and blend until smooth. When cupcakes have cooled, use a spoon or blunt knife to ice each one. Store in refrigerator.

Makes 12.

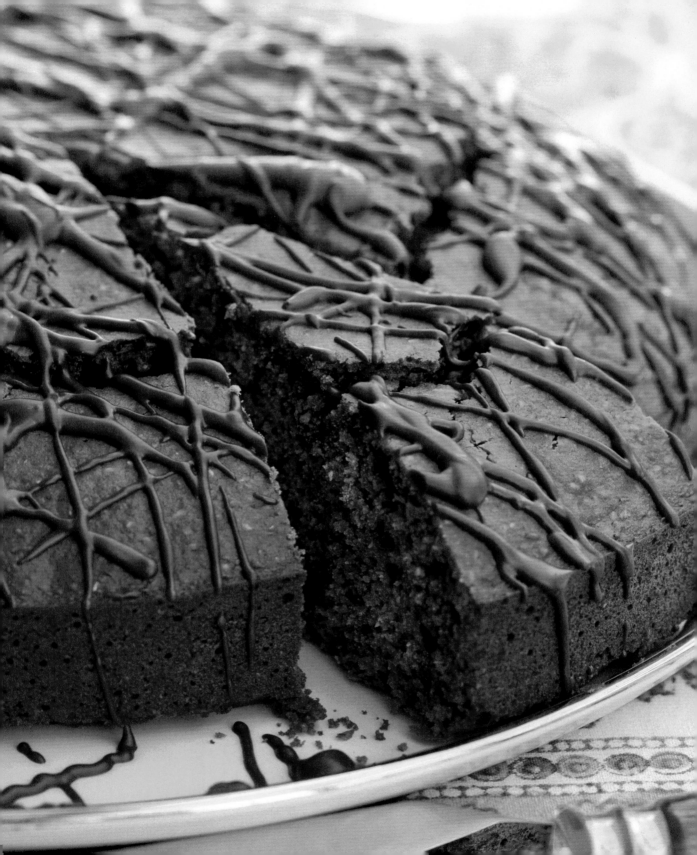

chocolate date cake

ingredients

cake

2 eggs

½ cup (125 ml) rice bran oil

160 g 70% dark chocolate

½ cup (150 g) honey

2 cups (320 g) wholemeal
(wholewheat) self-raising flour

1 cup (250 ml) milk

⅓ cup (80 ml) boiling water

1 cup (165 g) chopped dates

icing

70 g 70% dark chocolate

1 tablespoon honey

1 teaspoon rice bran oil

Preheat oven to 160°C (315°F) fan-forced.

Beat eggs and oil until creamy. Melt chocolate and stir in honey until dissolved. Mix chocolate mixture into the eggs and oil. Add flour and milk, alternating between the ingredients until they are combined. Add boiling water and mix well. Add chopped dates. Use your fingers to break them up and spread them evenly over the bowl, then stir into mixture.

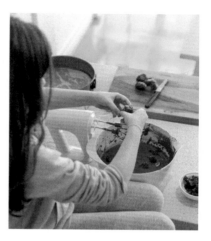

Grease a 24 cm round tin with oil and line the base with baking paper.

Bake for 40 to 45 minutes.

Leave cake to cool in tin for at least 20 minutes before removing and cooling on a cake rack.

To make the icing melt chocolate and stir in honey and oil. When the cake is cool, drizzle icing over the top of the cake.

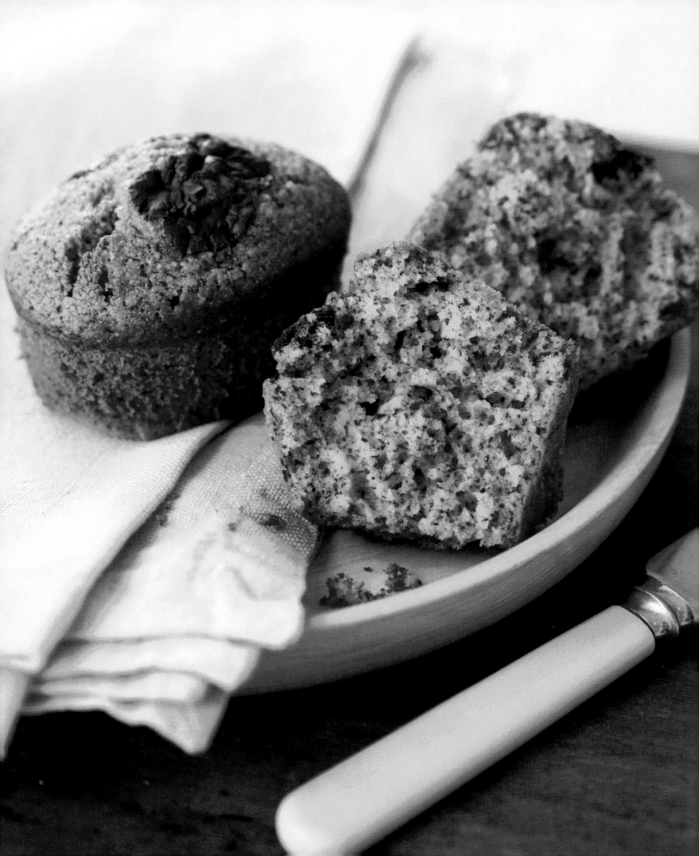

jaffa friands

ingredients

4 egg whites

½ cup (150 g) honey

½ cup (125 ml) rice bran oil

4 tablespoons orange juice

1 teaspoon finely grated orange rind

1 cup (110 g) almond meal

½ cup (80 g) wholemeal
(wholewheat) self-raising flour

¼ cup (25 g) grated 70% dark
chocolate, plus extra chopped
chocolate to garnish

Preheat oven to 160°C (315°F) fan-forced.

Whisk egg whites until fluffy and bubbles have formed on the top.
Dissolve honey in oil and add to the egg whites. Mix in orange juice
and orange rind, then mix in almond meal. Add flour and whisk for
a few minutes until mixture thickens (it will still be a little runny).
Mix in grated chocolate.

Grease a friand tin well with oil and cut oval shapes out of baking
paper to place on the base of each case to prevent sticking.

Pour mixture into friand cases, filling each one ¾ full. Chop up
some dark chocolate and place 4 or 5 small pieces on top of the
centre of each one.

Bake for 30 minutes.

Leave to cool completely in the tin.

Run a knife carefully around the edges of each friand to help lift
them out. Gently pull off baking paper.

Makes 8 to 10.

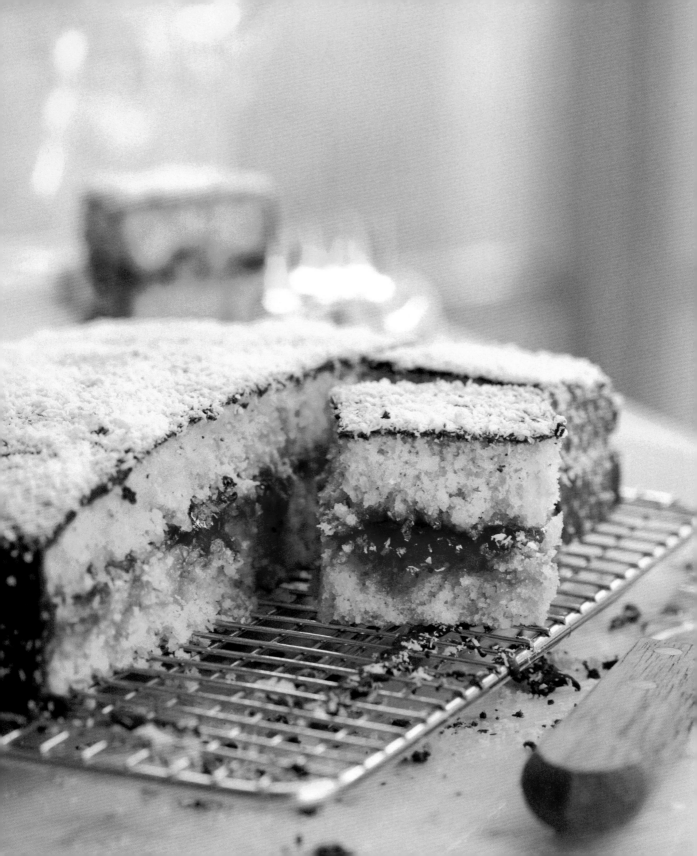

lamington cake

ingredients

cake

4 eggs

½ cup (150 g) honey

⅔ cup (165 ml) rice bran oil

1 vanilla bean

1 tablespoon boiling water

⅔ cup (110 g) wholemeal
  (wholewheat) self-raising flour

⅓ cup (30 g) desiccated coconut

4 tablespoons cornflour

125 g 100% strawberry jam

icing

150 g 70% dark chocolate

½ cup (50 g) desiccated coconut, for
  decoration

Preheat oven to 160°C (315°F) fan-forced.

Beat eggs until thick and fluffy. Add honey, oil, vanilla bean seeds and water to the eggs and mix until combined. (To extract seeds, cut vanilla bean lengthways and scrape out the seeds with a knife.)

In a separate bowl mix together flour, coconut and cornflour. Add egg mixture and combine.

Grease a lamington tin (23 cm × 32 cm) with oil and line the base with baking paper. Pour in mixture and bake for 20 minutes.

Leave cake to cool in tin for 20 minutes. Remove from tin and cool further on a cake rack.

Once the lamington cake has cooled slice it in half so you have 2 flat cakes. Spread strawberry jam over one half and place the other half on top.

Melt chocolate and use a spatula to cover the top and sides of the cake with chocolate, then sprinkle with coconut.

Hint: I use a teaspoon to sprinkle the coconut over the top of the lamington and my fingers to sprinkle the coconut over the sides.

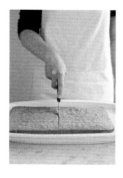 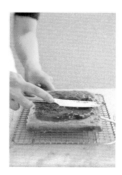 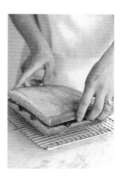 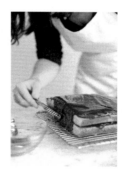 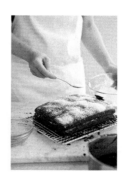

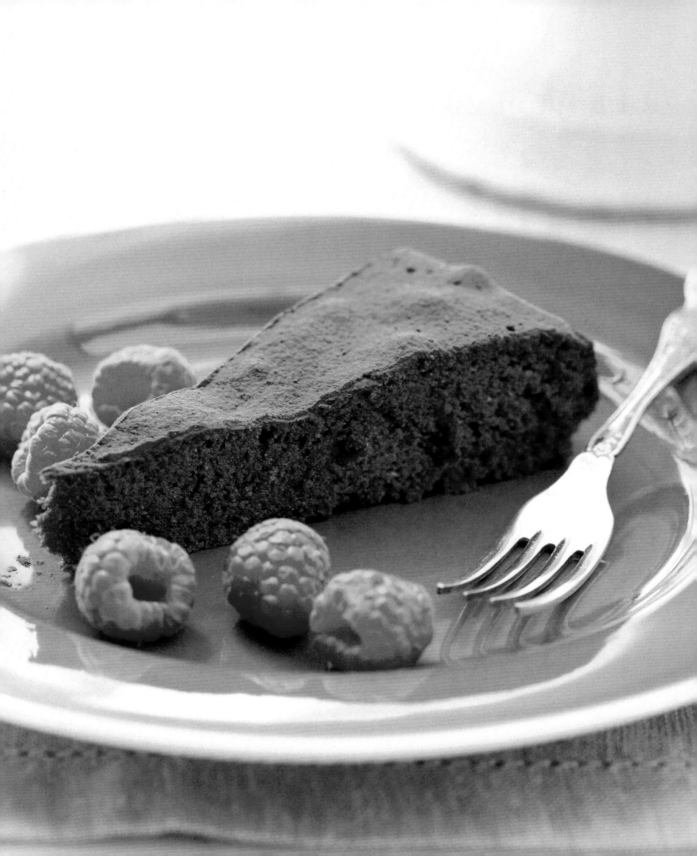

flourless chocolate cake

ingredients

4 eggs, separated
½ cup (125 ml) rice bran oil
160 g 70% dark chocolate
⅔ cup (190 g) honey
1½ cups (165 g) almond meal

Preheat oven to 160°C (315°F) fan-forced.

Beat egg whites until stiff.

In a separate bowl beat egg yolks and oil together. Melt chocolate and mix honey into chocolate until honey is dissolved. Add chocolate mixture to egg mixture and beat.

Mix almond meal into chocolate mixture, and then gently fold in egg whites until completely combined.

Grease a 25 cm springform tin with oil and line base with baking paper.

Pour in mixture and bake for 35 minutes.

Leave to cool in tin for at least 20 minutes. Remove and cool on a cake rack (run a knife around the outside of the cake to loosen it from the tin before removing).

Serve with fresh raspberries.

Hint: For a more professional look when entertaining guests, dust the cake with Dutch cocoa.

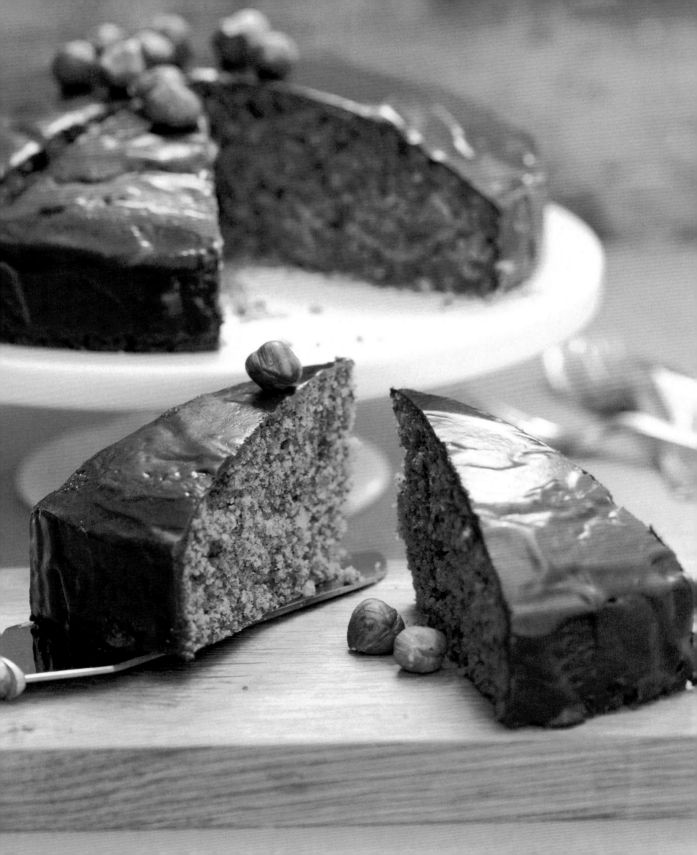

chocolate hazelnut cake

ingredients

cake

2 eggs

½ cup (125 ml) rice bran oil

½ cup (150 g) honey

½ cup (125 ml) orange juice

¾ cup (80 g) hazelnut meal

1 cup (160 g) wholemeal
(wholewheat) self-raising flour

⅓ cup (35 g) finely grated 70% dark
chocolate

icing

70 g 70% dark chocolate

1 tablespoon honey

2 teaspoons rice bran oil

hazelnuts for decorating

Preheat oven to 160°C (315°F) fan-forced.

Whisk together eggs, oil and honey. Add orange juice. Mix in hazelnut meal and flour until combined.

Add grated dark chocolate and mix.

Grease a 20 cm round tin with oil and line the base with baking paper. Pour in mixture and bake for 35 to 40 minutes.

Allow to cool for 20 minutes before removing and leaving to cool on a cake rack.

When cake has cooled prepare icing. Melt chocolate and stir in honey and oil. Mix until honey is dissolved. Use a blunt knife to ice the top and sides of the cake. Decorate with hazelnuts.

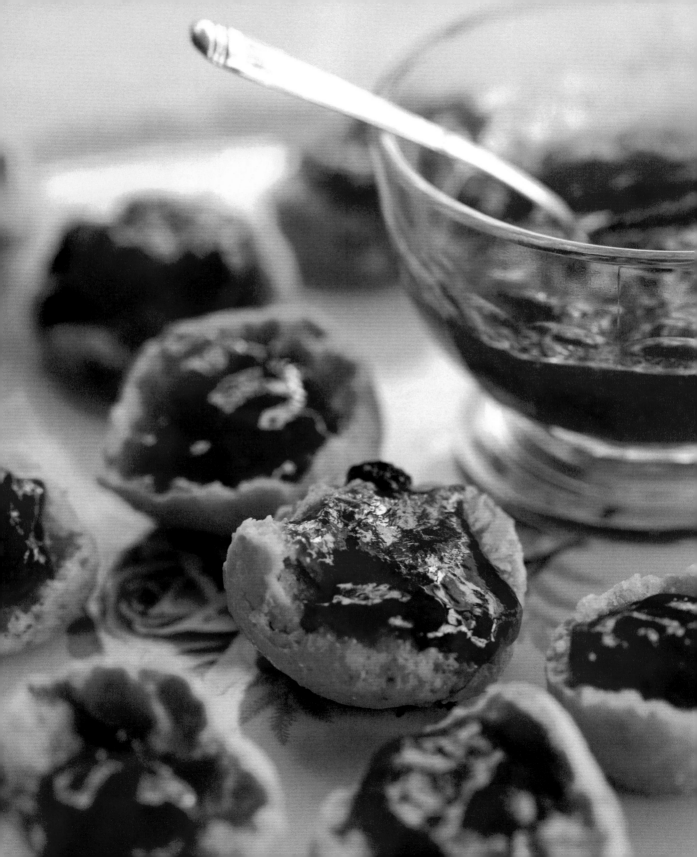

scones

ingredients

1¾ cups (280 g) wholemeal
    (wholewheat) self-raising flour

1 dessertspoon honey

¼ cup (60 ml) rice bran oil

¾ cup (185 ml) milk

Preheat oven to 220°C (425°F) fan-forced.

Place flour in a bowl, and make a well in the centre. Dissolve honey in oil and pour into the well, along with the milk. Use a blunt knife to stir mixture until a soft dough has formed.

You can make fruit scones by adding ½ cup of mixed dried fruit such as sultanas, apricots and sunflower seeds at this point. Place some flour on the bench and knead dough lightly. Use a 5 cm round cutter to cut out scones. Line a tray with baking paper and place scones close together on the tray.

Bake for 10 to 12 minutes or until the scones are golden.

Serve with 100% jam.

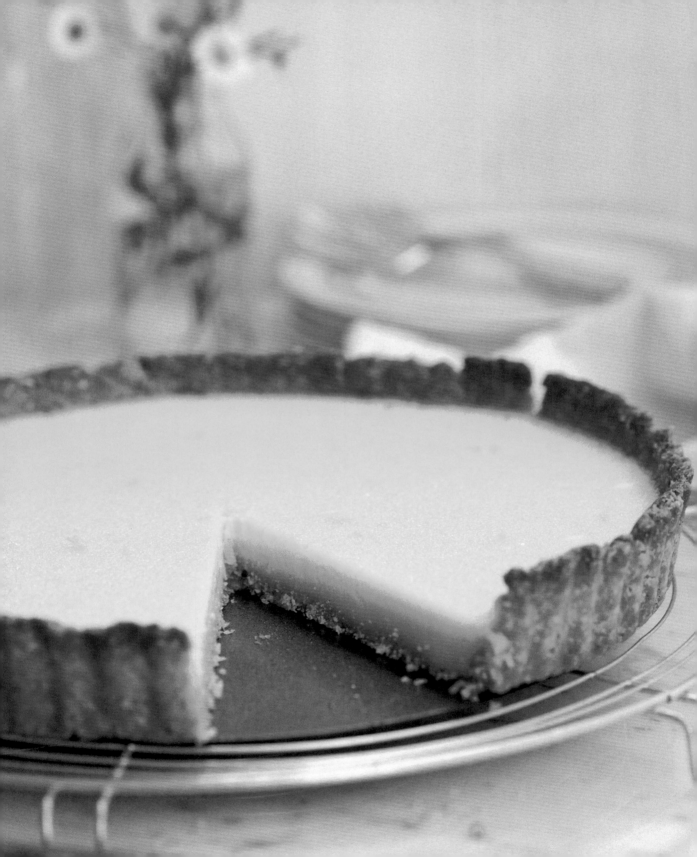

lemon tart

ingredients

pastry

2½ cups (400 g) wholemeal
  (wholewheat) plain flour

⅔ cup (165 ml) rice bran oil

¼ cup (75 g) honey

2 eggs

1 vanilla bean

2 tablespoons milk

filling

4 eggs

2 tablespoons rice bran oil

½ cup (150 g) honey

½ cup (125 ml) lemon juice

⅔ cup (165 ml) milk

2 tablespoons cornflour

Preheat oven to 200°C (390°F) fan-forced.

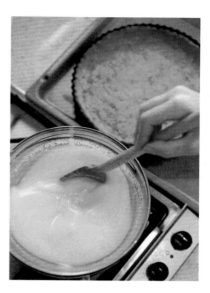

To prepare pastry refer to page 6, 'Making pastry'. Grease a 24 cm tart tin with oil. Place pastry in tart tin and refrigerate for 20 minutes. Remove from fridge and blind bake for 10 minutes. Remove baking paper and rice or baking beads. Allow the oven to cool to 160°C (315°F) and bake for a further 10 minutes.

To prepare filling, place a heatproof bowl over a saucepan

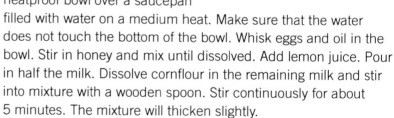

filled with water on a medium heat. Make sure that the water does not touch the bottom of the bowl. Whisk eggs and oil in the bowl. Stir in honey and mix until dissolved. Add lemon juice. Pour in half the milk. Dissolve cornflour in the remaining milk and stir into mixture with a wooden spoon. Stir continuously for about 5 minutes. The mixture will thicken slightly.

Reduce oven temperature to 140°C (285°F).

Pour filling into warm tart base and bake for a further 20 minutes or until filling sets. The centre can be slightly wobbly when shaken.

Refrigerate when cool.

Hint: If it's easier, whisk the eggs, oil, honey and lemon juice together before placing over the saucepan.

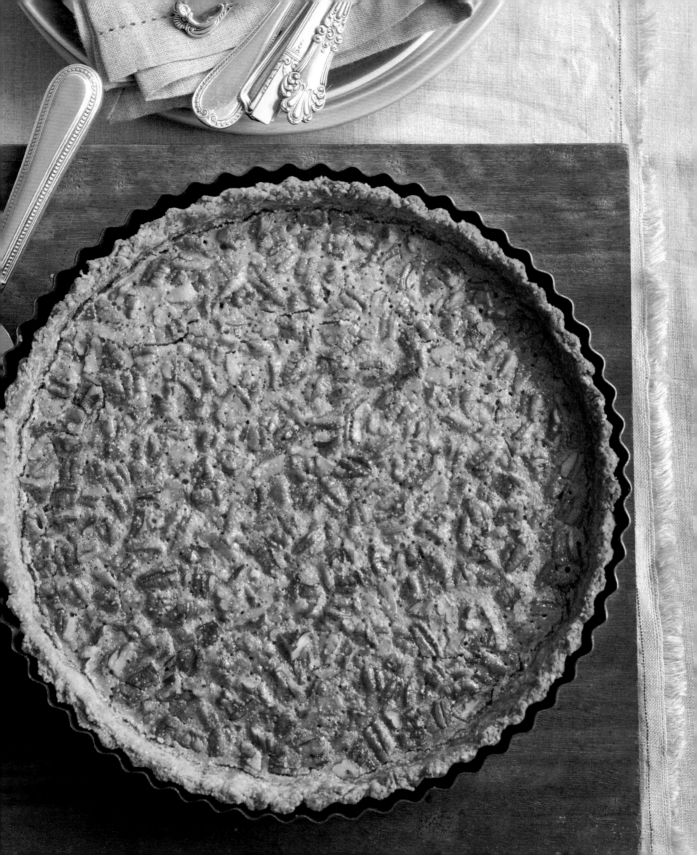

pecan tart

ingredients

pastry

2½ cups (400 g) wholemeal (wholewheat) plain flour

⅔ cup (165 ml) rice bran oil

¼ cup (75 g) honey

2 eggs

½ vanilla bean

2 tablespoons milk

filling

1½ cups (165 g) chopped pecans

2 eggs

½ cup (150 g) honey

⅓ cup (80 ml) rice bran oil

½ vanilla bean

3 tablespoons almond meal

Preheat oven to 200°C (390°F) fan-forced.

To prepare pastry refer to page 6, 'Making pastry'.

Grease a 24 cm tart tin with oil and press pastry into the base. Refrigerate for 20 minutes and then blind bake pastry for 10 minutes. Remove the baking beads and baking paper. Reduce oven heat to 160°C (315°F) and place the tart shell back in the oven for a further 10 minutes.

To prepare filling, chop pecan nuts and set aside.

Whisk together eggs, honey and oil. Scrape out seeds from the remaining half of the vanilla bean and mix in. Add almond meal and whisk until smooth.

Scatter chopped pecans evenly over the pastry base, then pour filling over pecans.

Reduce oven heat to 140°C (285°F) and bake for 35 to 40 minutes or until the filling sets.

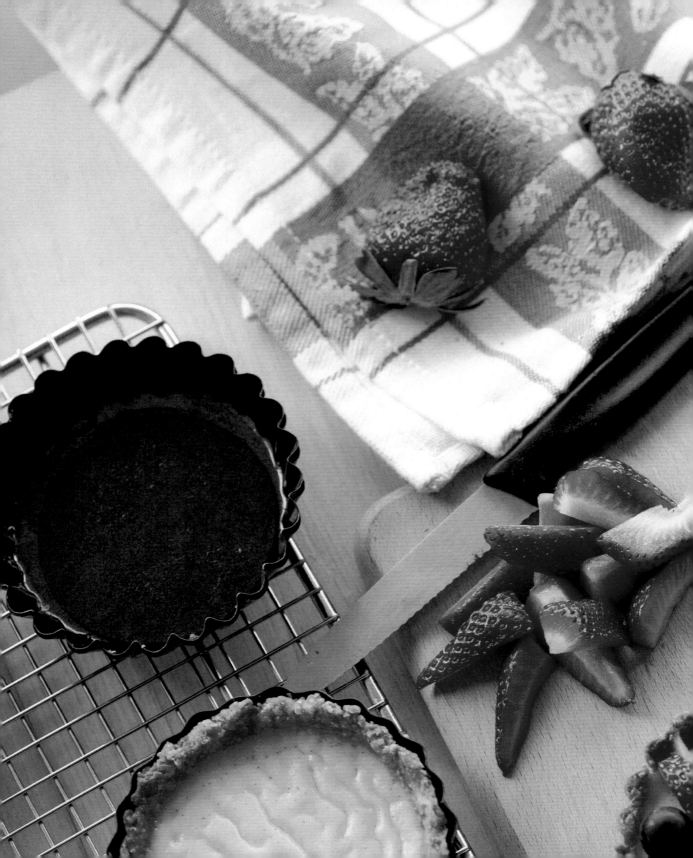

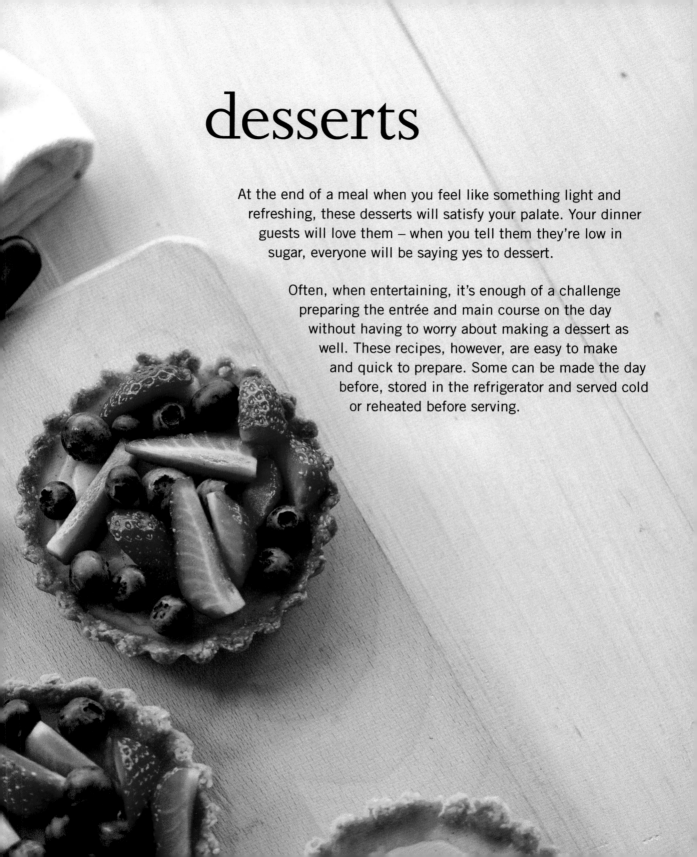

desserts

At the end of a meal when you feel like something light and refreshing, these desserts will satisfy your palate. Your dinner guests will love them – when you tell them they're low in sugar, everyone will be saying yes to dessert.

Often, when entertaining, it's enough of a challenge preparing the entrée and main course on the day without having to worry about making a dessert as well. These recipes, however, are easy to make and quick to prepare. Some can be made the day before, stored in the refrigerator and served cold or reheated before serving.

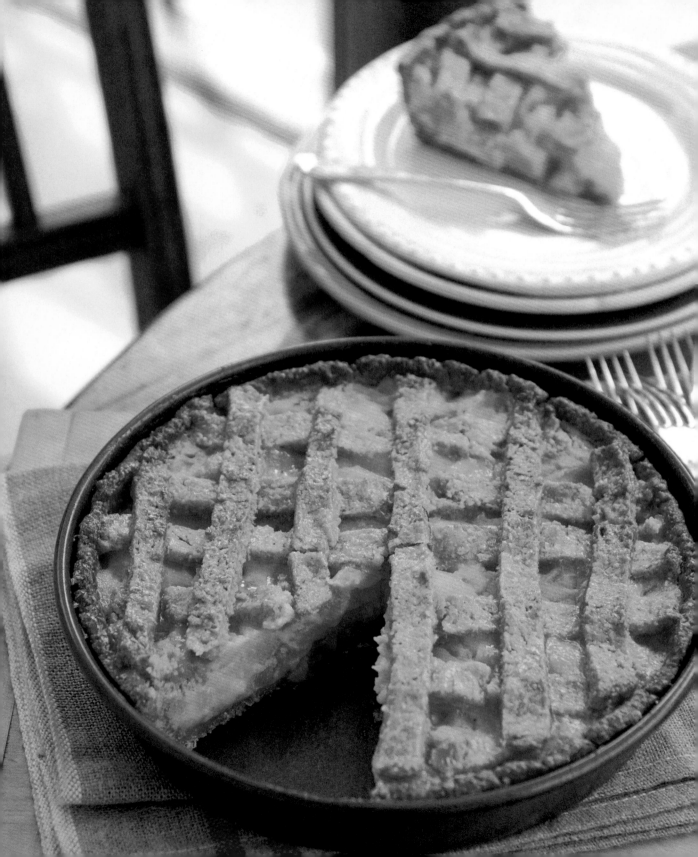

warm apple and frangipane pie

ingredients

pastry

2½ cups (400 g) wholemeal (wholewheat) plain flour

⅔ cup (165 ml) rice bran oil

¼ cup (75 g) honey

2 eggs

1 vanilla bean

2 tablespoons milk

2 tablespoons 100% apricot jam

filling

3 cups (670 g) cooked apples (fresh or tinned)

1 egg

½ cup (125 ml) rice bran oil

¼ cup (75 g) honey

½ cup (55 g) almond meal

Preheat oven to 200°C (390°F) fan-forced.

To prepare pastry see page 6, 'Making pastry'.

Grease a pie dish (24 cm) with oil and cover base and sides with pastry (there will be some left over). Refrigerate for 20 minutes and then blind bake for 10 minutes. Reduce oven temperature to 160°C (315°F).

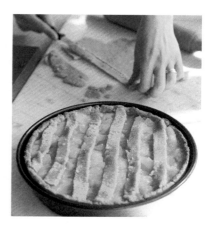

Remove baking beads and baking paper, allow oven to cool and bake for a further 10 minutes.

Set aside the remaining pastry mix for the top of the pie.

To cook apples, place the sliced apples in a saucepan with water. Bring to the boil then reduce heat to low and simmer for 15 minutes. Drain well. (If using tinned apples make sure you buy a brand with no added sugar.)

To prepare the frangipane filling whisk egg, oil and honey in a bowl and mix in almond meal. Place in the fridge while the pastry is cooking. Pour frangipane mix over the base of the pie and then spread the cooked apples over the top.

Roll out the remaining pastry and cut into strips to make a crisscross shape on top. If they break when transferring to the top of the pie, just press them together again.

Bake for 40 minutes on 160°C (315°F).

Warm the apricot jam in a saucepan on a low heat and press through a strainer with a spoon to remove any lumps. Brush the top of the pie with the jam.

Serve warm.

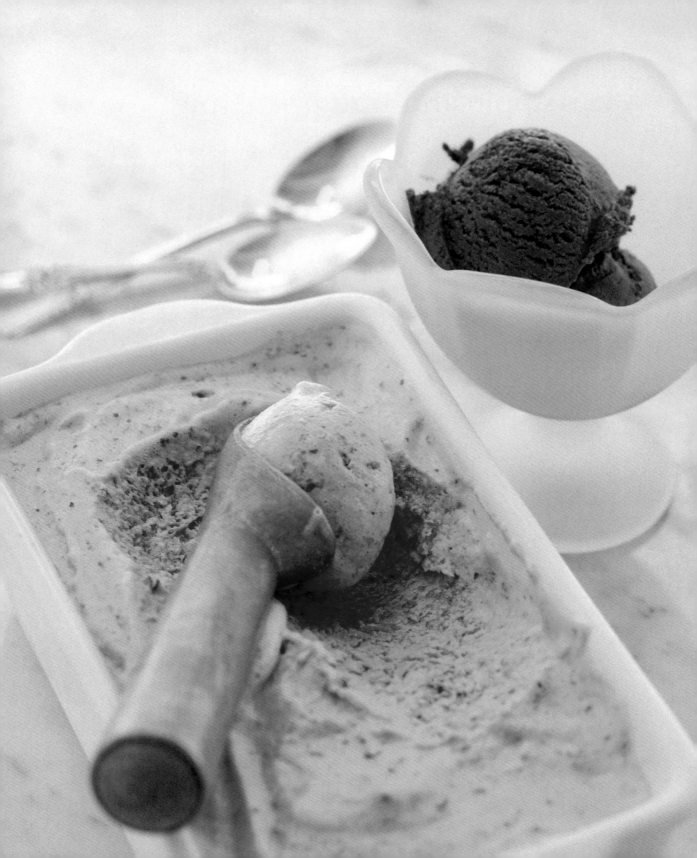

strawberry ice-cream

ingredients
250 g fresh strawberries
¼ cup (75 g) honey
2 egg whites

Prepare this dish the day before serving.

Blend or mash strawberries and place in a bowl with the honey and egg whites.

Use an electric beater to beat all ingredients together for 10 minutes or until stiff.

Transfer to a container and place in the freezer.

chocolate ice-cream

ingredients
6 egg whites
80 g 70% dark chocolate
⅓ cup (95 g) honey
2 tablespoons milk

Prepare this dish the day before serving.

Beat egg whites until stiff.

Melt chocolate. Add honey and stir until dissolved. Mix in milk. Gently fold chocolate mixture into the egg whites.

Place in a container and freeze.

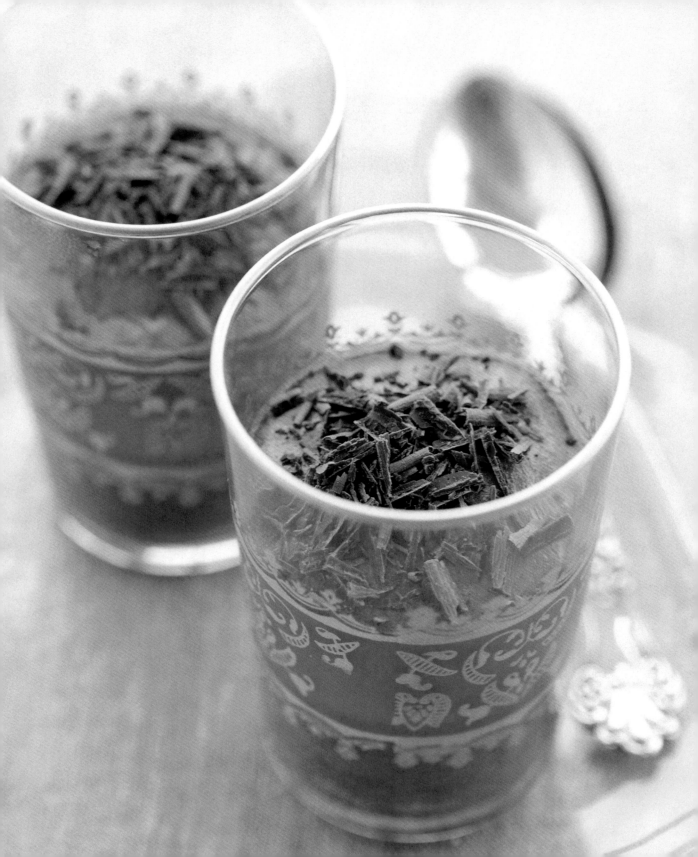

chocolate mousse

ingredients

4 eggs

2 egg whites

120 g 70% dark chocolate

⅓ cup (95 g) honey

1½ tablespoons orange juice

Beat egg whites until stiff.

In a separate bowl beat egg yolks. Melt chocolate and add honey, stirring until dissolved. Combine the chocolate mixture with the egg yolks and stir in orange juice.

Gently fold the mixture into the egg whites.

Place in either individual serving dishes or a large bowl and leave mousse to set in the fridge. Make mousse the day before serving to allow plenty of time for it to set.

To serve, grate some dark chocolate and sprinkle over the top and serve with berries.

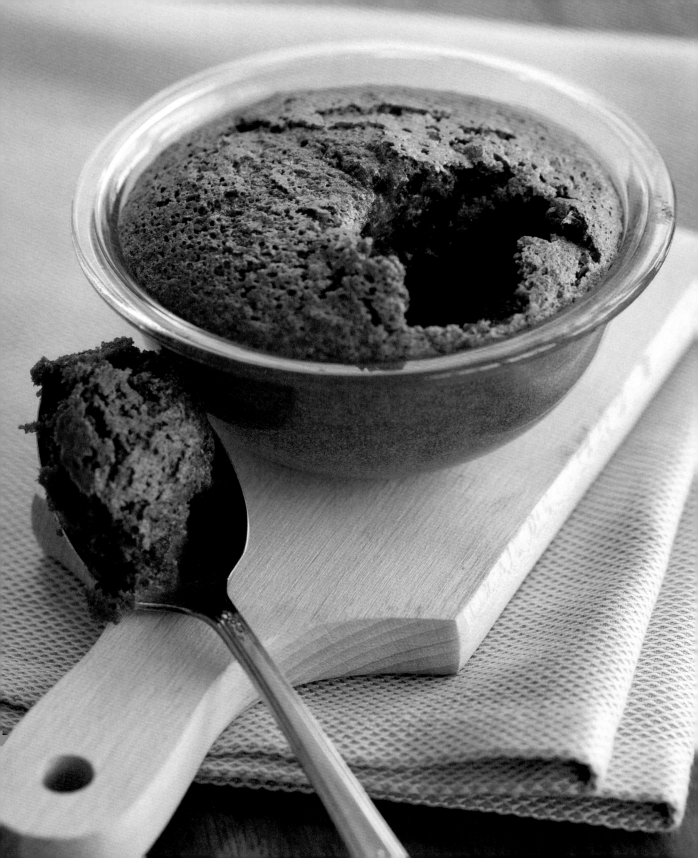

chocolate pudding

ingredients

2 eggs, separated

75 g 70% dark chocolate

½ cup (150 g) honey

1 tablespoon rice bran oil

½ cup (80 g) wholemeal
   (wholewheat) self-raising flour

⅔ cup (165 ml) milk

Preheat oven to 170°C (335°F) fan-forced.

Beat egg whites until stiff.

Melt chocolate and add honey. Stir until dissolved. Beat egg yolks and oil together then stir in chocolate mixture. Add flour and milk. Gently fold in egg whites.

Pour into baking dishes or 8 cm ramekins.

Bake for 12 to 15 minutes (if using a larger dish, you may need to bake your pudding for a few extra minutes).

Serve straight from the oven.

Serves 8.

Hint: If you like your pudding nice and gooey in the centre, cook for 12 minutes.

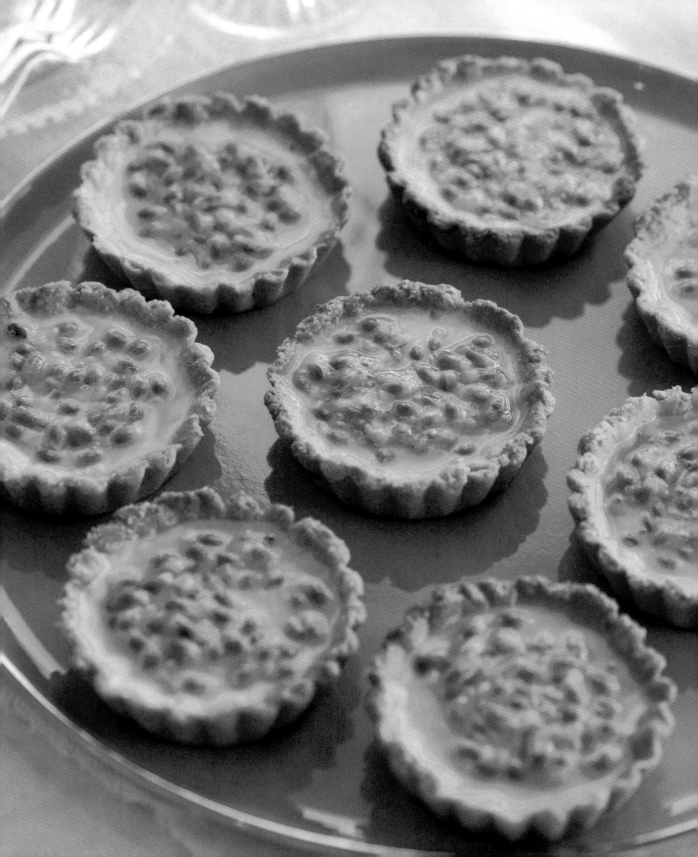

passionfruit tarts

ingredients

pastry

1¼ cups (200 g) wholemeal
  (wholewheat) plain flour

¼ cup (40 g) wholemeal
  (wholewheat) self-raising flour

⅓ cup (80 ml) rice bran oil

¼ cup (75 g) honey

1 egg

1 teaspoon finely grated orange rind

1 tablespoon milk

custard filling

1 vanilla bean

1 cup (250 ml) milk

1 tablespoon cornflour

1 egg

1 egg yolk

1½ tablespooons honey

5 passionfruits

Preheat oven to 200°C (390°F) fan-forced.

To prepare pastry refer to page 6, 'Making pastry'.

Grease 10, 8 cm tart tins with oil. Press pastry into tart tins and refrigerate for 20 minutes. Blind bake tart shells for 10 minutes. Remove the baking paper and rice or baking beads from the pastry and let the oven cool to 160°C (315°F) before placing tarts back in the oven for a further 5 minutes.

Begin to prepare the custard at this point. Cut vanilla bean lengthways and place it in a saucepan with ¾ of the milk. Dissolve cornflour in the remaining milk and set aside. In a separate bowl whisk egg, extra egg yolk and honey. When milk begins to simmer turn the heat to medium low, remove vanilla bean and stir in egg mixture and cornflour mixture. Stir continuously for 2 to 3 minutes (the custard will thicken slightly).

Remove saucepan from the stove and mix in the pulp of 1 passionfruit.

Reduce the oven temperature to 140°C (285°F).

Fill each tart with the custard mix and place back in the oven for roughly 10 to 15 minutes, until the custard centre has set. The amount of time this takes will depend on how thick the custard becomes in the saucepan. Allow to cool.

Remove pulp from remaining passionfruits, pour over each of the tarts and serve. Store in the refrigerator.

Makes 10.

Hint: If the custard becomes lumpy, pass it through a strainer.

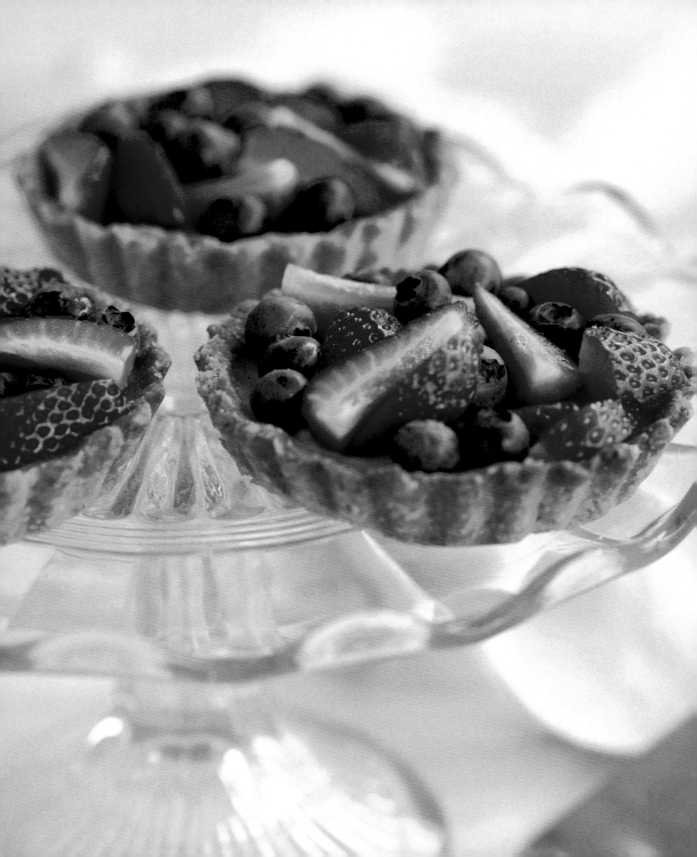

berry and custard tarts

ingredients

pastry
2½ cups (400 g) wholemeal (wholewheat) plain flour

⅔ cup (165 ml) rice bran oil

¼ cup (75 g) honey

2 eggs

1 vanilla bean

2 tablespoons milk

custard filling
2 cups (500 ml) milk

2 tablespoons cornflour

1 vanilla bean

2 eggs

2 egg yolks

3 tablespoons honey

Preheat oven to 200°C (390°F) fan-forced.

To prepare pastry refer to page 6, 'Making pastry'.

Grease 8, 10 cm tart tins with oil and press pastry into each tart tin. Refrigerate for 20 minutes and then blind bake for 10 minutes. Remove the baking paper and rice or baking beads and allow the oven to cool to 160°C (315°F) before baking for a further 5 minutes.

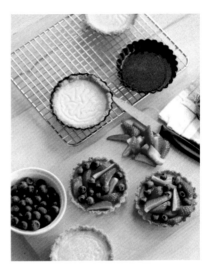

To prepare custard, pour milk into a saucepan, leaving ¼ cup of milk for later. Cut vanilla bean lengthways and scrape the seeds into the milk.

In a separate bowl whisk eggs, extra yolks and honey. Dissolve cornflour in the remaining milk. Heat milk until it begins to simmer, then turn the heat to medium low. Pour egg mixture and cornflour into the milk and stir continuously for 2 to 3 minutes. The custard will thicken slightly (if it becomes lumpy, pass it through a strainer).

Reduce the oven temperature to 140°C (285°F). While tarts are still hot fill them with custard (this will prevent the mixture from leaking out of the tart shell). Bake for 20 minutes or until the custard has set. Allow to cool.

To serve, place some fresh blueberries and sliced strawberries over the top of each tart.

Makes 10.

apple crumble

ingredients

1½ cups (335 g) sliced cooked apples (fresh or tinned)

¼ cup (75 g) honey

½ cup (125 ml) rice bran oil

½ teaspoon cinnamon

½ cup (50 g) desiccated coconut

½ cup (80 g) wholemeal (wholewheat) self-raising flour

½ cup (60 g) slivered almonds

Preheat oven to 160°C (315°F) fan-forced.

To prepare the cooked apples, place the sliced apples in a saucepan with some water. Bring to the boil then reduce heat to low and simmer for 10 minutes. Drain well and cover the base of the baking dish with the sliced apples. (If using tinned apples, make sure they are 100% apples with no added sugar.)

To prepare crumble, mix honey and oil together and add cinnamon. Mix in coconut, flour and slivered almonds.

Spread crumble mixture over the apples with a spoon until all the apples are covered.

Bake for 30 minutes or until the crumble is golden.

Serves 6 to 8.

Hint: If using a larger baking dish, just double the above quantities.

banana fritters

ingredients

2 tablespoons desiccated coconut

1 cup (160 g) wholemeal
   (wholewheat) self-raising flour

⅔ cup (165 ml) milk

⅓ cup (80 ml) cold water

3 teaspoons honey

1 tablespoon boiling water

3 bananas

cinnamon for dusting

rice bran oil for frying

To prepare the batter place coconut and flour in a bowl. Using a whisk or spoon slowly mix in the milk a little at a time. Add cold water a little at a time until the batter is nice and smooth. In a separate bowl dissolve honey in boiling water. Add to batter and mix until combined.

Slice 3 bananas in half lengthways and then again in half on a diagonal.

Dust each banana slice with cinnamon and then dip into the batter.

Pour enough oil into the frying pan to cover the base, and heat on high. To test if frying pan is hot enough place a drop of batter into the pan; if the oil bubbles around the batter it is ready to use.

Place the banana fritters into the oil. Don't over-crowd the frying pan. When the fritters have browned on one side (1 to 2 minutes) flip them over and brown the other side. Remove and place on paper towel to remove any excess oil.

Serve warm.

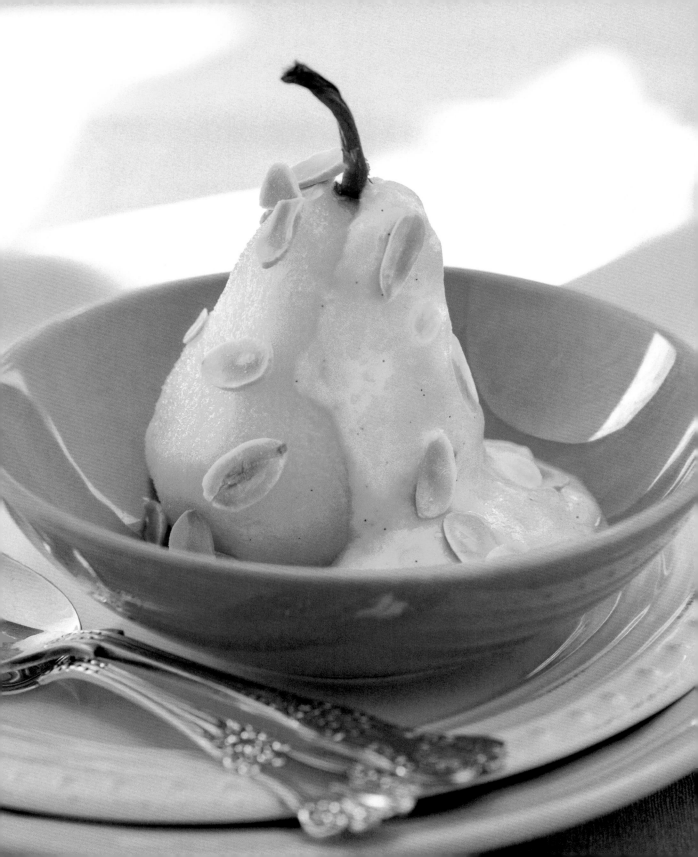

poached pears with custard

ingredients

4 ripe pears

4 cups (1 L) water

⅓ cup (95 g) honey

½ vanilla bean

1 sliver orange rind

1 sliver lemon rind

½ cup (55 g) flaked almonds

custard

1 cup (250 ml) milk

½ vanilla bean

2 teaspoons cornflour

1 egg

1 egg yolk

1½ tablespoons honey

Peel the skin of 4 firm, ripe pears, leaving them whole. Use a knife to trim some of the core from the base so it sits flat. Place water and honey in a saucepan over a medium heat. Add one half of the vanilla bean (cut vanilla bean lengthways). Add a sliver of orange and lemon rind.

When the water begins to simmer turn heat to low and place pears into the saucepan. Leave to simmer for 15 to 18 minutes. When cooked remove the pears from the liquid.

Toast almond flakes in the oven for 8 to10 minutes at 180°C (350°F).

To prepare the custard, place milk in a saucepan, leaving a little aside for later.

Add seeds from the remaining half of the vanilla bean to the milk and heat.

In a separate bowl whisk egg, egg yolk and honey together. Dissolve cornflour in the remaining milk and whisk into the egg mixture.

When the milk is starting to bubble around the edges turn the heat to medium and pour in the egg mixture, stirring continuously with a wooden spoon. The mixture will begin to thicken within 2 to 3 minutes. Remove from heat and continue to stir (keep in mind that if the heat is too high the eggs will scramble, and if it's too low the custard won't thicken).

Place the custard in a jug or bowl to cool a little.

To serve stand each pear in a serving dish, pour the custard over it and sprinkle with toasted almond flakes.

Serves 4.

Hint: If the custard becomes a little lumpy, place through a strainer and you will have a nice smooth custard.

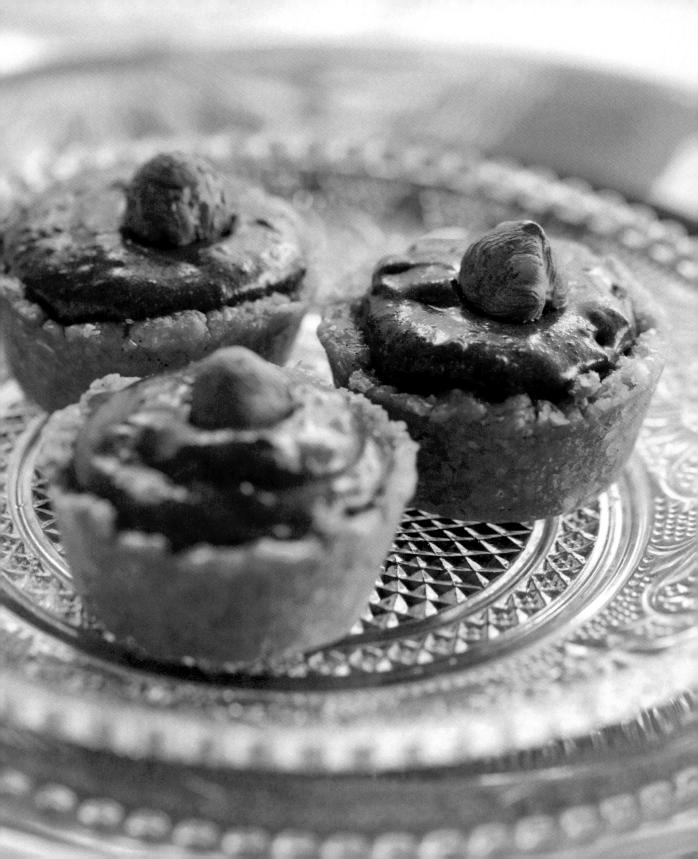

chocolate hazelnut mousse tarts

ingredients

pastry

2½ cups (400 g) wholemeal (wholewheat) plain flour

⅔ cup (165 ml) rice bran oil

¼ cup (75 g) honey

2 eggs

1 vanilla bean

2 tablespoons milk

filling

4 eggs, separated

120 g 70% dark chocolate

⅓ cup (95 g) honey

½ cup (65 g) hazelnuts

24 hazelnuts for decoration

Preheat oven to 200°C (390°F) fan-forced.

To prepare pastry refer to page 6, 'Making pastry'.

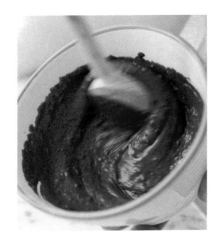

Grease mini muffin tins with oil. Roll out pastry and cut circles out to place in each muffin case. When placing pastry in the cases, press pastry into the sides first and then into the base of the cases. Cut away any excess pastry with a knife. Refrigerate for 20 minutes.

Use a fork to place little holes in the pastry bases (don't go all the way through the pastry) and bake uncovered for 5 minutes. Remove from oven, reduce the oven temperature to 160°C (315°F), then return tins to the oven and bake for a further 10 minutes.

To prepare chocolate hazelnut mousse, beat egg whites until stiff and set aside. Melt chocolate and stir in honey. In a separate bowl beat egg yolks and add chocolate mixture.

Place hazelnuts in a food processor and blend to fine pieces. Add hazelnuts to the chocolate mixture. Gently fold in egg whites until mixed through.

Refrigerate to set.

When tart shells have cooled, fill with mousse and place a hazelnut on top. Store in the fridge until you are ready to serve.

Makes 24.

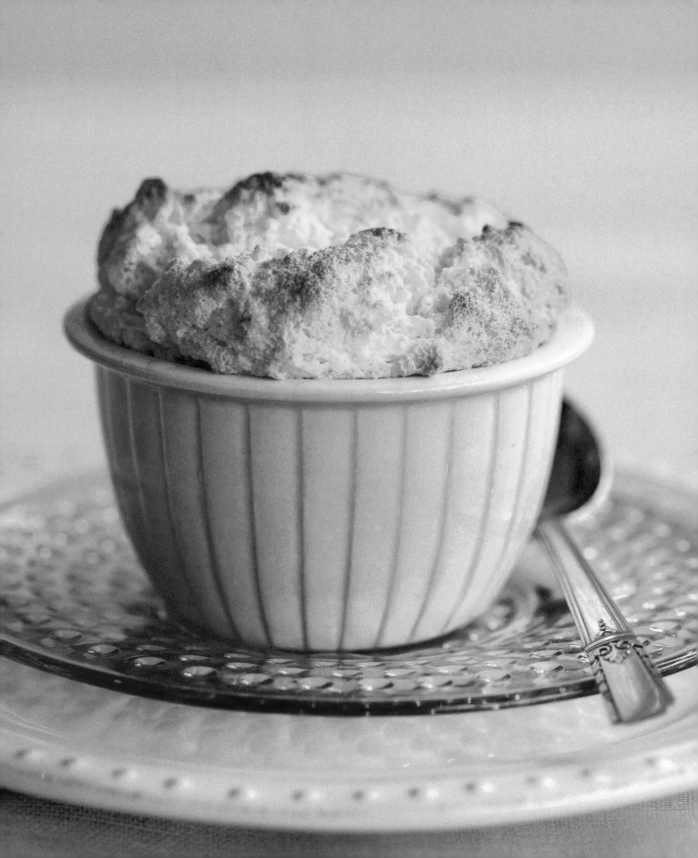

orange and passionfruit soufflé

ingredients

4 egg whites

2 egg yolks

¼ cup (75 g) honey

¼ teaspoon finely grated orange rind

¼ cup (60 ml) orange juice

¼ cup (60 ml) passionfruit juice
  (approximately 3–4 passionfruits)

2 tablespoons wholemeal
  (wholewheat) plain flour

Preheat oven to 160°C (315°F) fan-forced.

Beat egg whites until stiff.

In a separate bowl beat together egg yolks and honey. Add orange rind – use the back of a spoon to rub the rind against the side of the bowl to make sure it is dissolved.

Add orange juice to the egg yolks. Press passionfruit pulp through a strainer with a spoon to extract the juice. Discard seeds and add juice to the yolk mixture. Mix in flour.

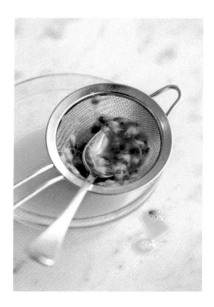

Gently fold egg whites into the mixture until completely combined.

Grease six 8 cm ramekin dishes with oil inside the dish and around the rim and then fill to the brim with mixture.

Bake for 15 to 20 minutes. Check after 15 minutes by placing a skewer into the centre of one. It's okay if the skewer has mixture on it, but you don't want it to be runny.

Serve straight from the oven.

Serves 6.

pizza with chocolate and strawberries

ingredients

pizza base

1¾ cups (280 g) wholemeal
   (wholewheat) self-raising flour

¼ cup (60 ml) rice bran oil

⅔ cup (165 ml) boiling water

2 teaspoons honey

topping

100 g 70% dark chocolate

1 tablespoon honey

250 g strawberries

Preheat oven to 210°C (410°F) fan-forced.

Place flour in a bowl, making a well in the centre. Add oil to the centre. Add honey to the boiled water, stir until dissolved then mix into flour. Using a blunt knife stir until combined. Knead for 2 to 3 minutes and then roll out the dough. Halve the dough and roll each half into 2 thin circles.

Brush each pizza base with oil and bake for 12 minutes or until golden (the bottom tray may need an extra 2 minutes).

Melt chocolate. Add honey and mix until dissolved.

Spread chocolate over each base and scatter with sliced strawberries.

Serve warm.

Makes 2.

sticky date cake

ingredients

1½ cups (315 g) dates

1¼ cups (310 ml) boiling water

1 teaspoon bi-carb soda

¼ cup (60 ml) rice bran oil

½ cup (150 g) honey

2 eggs

2 tablespoons desiccated coconut

1 cup (160 g) wholemeal
  (wholewheat) self-raising flour

Preheat oven to 160°C (315°F) fan-forced.

Place dates in a bowl and cover with boiling water. Add bi-carb soda and leave to stand for 5 to 10 minutes.

Place oil, honey and eggs in a food processor and blend. Add dates and water and pulse for about 30 seconds.

Add coconut and flour and pulse until mixed through.

Grease a round 20 cm tin with oil and line the base with baking paper. Pour mixture into the tin and bake for 55 minutes or until the skewer comes out clean. It's okay if there's a little mixture on the skewer, as long as it's not runny.

Leave to cool in the tin for 15 minutes. Serve warm with custard (see page 109) and fresh berries.

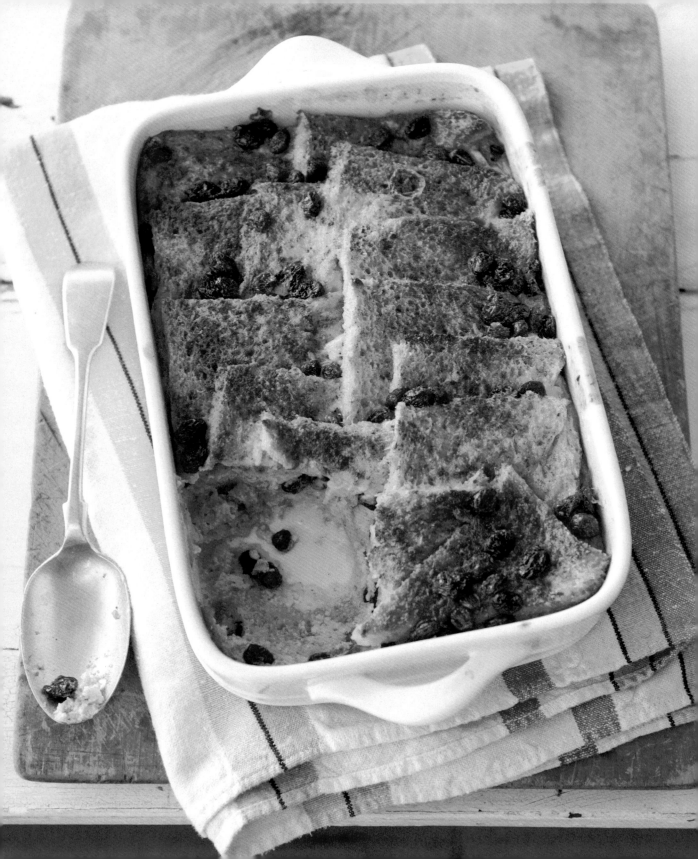

bread and butter pudding

ingredients

12 to 15 slices wholemeal
   (wholewheat) bread (toast slices)
rice bran oil for brushing
cinnamon for dusting
¾ cup (105 g) sultanas

custard

3 cups (750 ml) milk
1 vanilla bean
3 eggs
3 egg yolks
4½ tablespoons honey

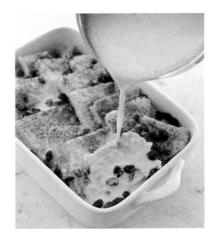

Preheat oven to 140°C (285°F) fan-forced.

Trim crusts off bread and slice into triangles. Brush each side with oil and spread ⅓ of the bread across the base of the baking dish. Sprinkle with cinnamon and then with ⅓ of the sultanas. Repeat the process for the next 2 layers (if using a lower dish, make 2 layers).

To prepare custard, heat milk with vanilla bean seeds until bubbles form around the edge; do not boil. (To extract seeds, cut vanilla bean lengthways and scrape out the seeds with a knife.) In a separate bowl whisk eggs, egg yolks and honey together. Turn the heat to low and pour in egg mixture. Stir continuously for 3 to 4 minutes. Remove any clumps of vanilla bean seeds with a strainer or spoon.

Pour custard over the bread in the baking dish and leave to stand for 10 minutes so the bread can absorb the custard. Gently press your hands over the bread, before placing in the oven.

Bake for 45 to 50 minutes or until set.

Serve warm.

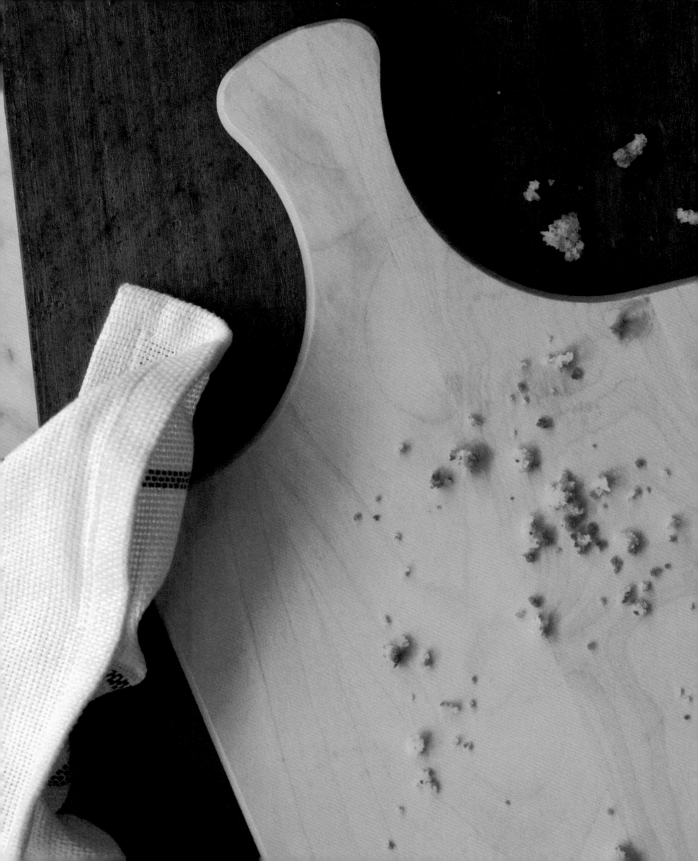

index